ELITE GOURMET AIR FRYER COOKBOOK

EFFORTLESS AIR FRYER RECIPES FOR BEGINNERS AND ADVANCED USERS

BOBBY MILLER

CONTENTS

INTRODUCTION

How air frying works

Have you ever seen one of those money machines, where someone steps inside a cylinder, closes the door, and air starts flowing up from the bottom with money flying through the air?

An air fryer is kind of like one of those money machines. When you put your food into the air fryer and close it, hot air circulates around the food and begins to cook it. The temperature of the air fryer and the type of food you're cooking will help determine the amount of time you need to cook your recipe.

The big difference between air frying and traditional deep frying is that air fryers require minimal to no oil to cook the food. The hot air circulating around the food helps to impart that crisp texture instead of the oil involved in deep frying.

A few other technologically advanced mechanisms are involved, but this is the gist of how air frying works. If you're familiar with convection ovens, where hot air is circulated (as opposed to conventional ovens, where the heating element is on the bottom), you'll feel right at home with air frying. An air fryer is essentially a compact convection oven.

If you want to get a bit more science based, what's actually happening from a chemical perspective when food is cooked in an air fryer is something called the Maillard reaction. The Maillard reaction is often referred to as "non-enzymatic browning," or basically a reaction that happens between sugars and amino acids in a recipe that result in the end product taking on a new flavor, texture, and color.

Seeing the benefits of air frying

Air frying is not only a healthier way to cook some more decadent recipes, but it's also efficient. Many popular models of air fryers claim that using an air fryer instead of a deep fryer can lower the fat of the dish by over 75 percent. This actually makes sense when you think about. Let's say you're going to make homemade fried chicken. If you were to use the deep-frying method of cooking, you'd traditionally need more than 3 cups of oil to cover the chicken to allow the cooking to ensue. On the other hand, if you were to use the air frying method, you'd need less than a tablespoon of oil.

Here are a few other benefits of air frying:

➢ **Air fryers can promote weight loss (for certain individuals).**

For individuals who currently have a highly processed diet filled with deep-fried foods, switching to air frying will certainly help with reducing caloric intake. A reduction in caloric intake will inevitably result in weight loss.

➢ **Air fryers can increase consumption of healthy foods, like fish, shrimp, and produce.**

Eating seafood at least twice a week, as well as increasing your consumption of fruits and vegetables, is highly recommended. If you struggle with getting your family to eat more of these foods on a regular basis, then air frying may be the best way to change their appetites (and minds!).

Not only can you put a light crunchy coating of heart-healthy nuts on some of your fried seafood favorites and cook them in the air fryer, but you can do the same with new herbs, spices, and vegetables! This is a great way to explore new vegetables and flavors in your kitchen, too.

➢ **Air fryers are safer (for the most part) than deep fryers.**

Deep frying can cause splatters of exceptionally hot oil all over your kitchen. Air fryers get super-hot as well, but they don't splatter in the same way a deep fryer does.

As long as you practice important safety measures when taking foods in and out of your fryer (for example, don't put your hands on the fryer basket), you can feel secure in using your fryer.

➢ **Air fryers can reduce the risk of potentially harmful agents on certain foods.**

A compound called *acrylamide* naturally forms on carbohydrate-rich foods (those traditionally deep-fried foods like french fries, breaded meats, and so on) when cooked at high temperatures. Some studies have found an association between acrylamide and cancer. The jury's still out on whether acrylamide actually *causes* cancer. What you need to know is that air frying is associated with a *decreased* amount of this compound as compared to deep frying, but some may still be present. We firmly believe in balance and moderation. We wouldn't recommend you eat french fries (even air-fried ones) daily.

➢ **Air fryers can reduce the risk of preventable diseases affected by diet and nutrition.**

This varies depending on many factors like your genetics and current lifestyle habits (such as nutrition and exercise). That said, if your diet is heavy in processed, fried foods, the air fryer may just be the ticket to enjoying the foods you crave in a new, exciting, and healthier way. Not only can you modify the amount of sodium in your recipes and use more fresh herbs and spices to give flavor to the food instead of salt, but you can also increase the fiber in your diet while including more plants in your meal plan.

Using Your Elite Gourmet Air Fryer

Each make and model of air fryer has its own instructions, but air fryers don't require extensive knowledge to operate. We recommend that you start by reading the manual that came with your Elite Gourmet air fryer and getting to know your particular machine.

With that said, here are a few basic steps that work for Your Elite Gourmet Air Fryer:

1. Clean the air fryer basket and accessories with hot soapy water and dry with a dish towel before use.
2. Plug in your air fryer and preheat it.

   This allows the machine time to get to temperature before you actually put the recipe inside.
3. Select Air Fry as the function.
4. Place your food on the wire rack or trivet, securely seal or close the drawer, and begin to air fry.
5. Check the food as applicable, following the recipe instructions.
6. When cooking completes, press Cancel and unplug the air fryer.

Caring for Your Elite Gourmet Air Fryer

You don't have to invest in any specific detergent or cleanser to keep your Elite Gourmet air fryer smelling like new. Use this section as your guide to keep your new kitchen appliance in tip-top shape so you can use it for years to come. Cleaning your Elite Gourmet air fryer is actually a really simple task. With a little elbow grease, some regular dish detergent, and hot water, your air fryer will come back to life, even with the toughest of buildup.

We've experimented with various makes and models and had our fair share of epic disasters in our air fryers, but guess what? After letting the basket and/or tray cool, we were easily able to get the buildup off with a regular kitchen sponge and hot soapy water.

Plus, even when switching between seafood and a decadent dessert, the air fryer doesn't require a deep clean.

Wipe down the outside of your fryer after each use. A hot, soapy towel is all that's necessary. This helps get off any grease or food particles that may have latched on during cooking.

Your Elite Gourmet air fryer manual may say that the parts to wash are dishwasher safe, but we recommend that you hand wash them instead. Why? Because hand washing will keep your air fryer in better shape than putting it through the wear and tear of the dishwasher. Just spend 5 minutes to give it a thorough hand wash after each use, and you'll have a properly working air fryer for years to come.

Appetizers And Snacks

Spinach Cups

Servings: 30

Cooking Time: 5 Minutes

Ingredients:

- 1 6-ounce can crabmeat, drained to yield ⅓ cup meat
- ¼ cup frozen spinach, thawed, drained, and chopped
- 1 clove garlic, minced
- ½ cup grated Parmesan cheese
- 3 tablespoons plain yogurt
- ¼ teaspoon lemon juice
- ½ teaspoon Worcestershire sauce
- 30 mini phyllo shells (2 boxes of 15 each), thawed
- cooking spray

Directions:

1. Remove any bits of shell that might remain in the crabmeat.
2. Mix crabmeat, spinach, garlic, and cheese together.
3. Stir in the yogurt, lemon juice, and Worcestershire sauce and mix well.
4. Spoon a teaspoon of filling into each phyllo shell.
5. Spray air fryer basket and arrange half the shells in the basket.
6. Cook at 390°F for 5minutes.
7. Repeat with remaining shells.

Cheeseburger Slider Pockets

Servings: 4

Cooking Time: 13 Minutes

Ingredients:

- 1 pound extra lean ground beef
- 2 teaspoons steak seasoning
- 2 tablespoons Worcestershire sauce
- 8 ounces Cheddar cheese
- ⅓ cup ketchup
- ¼ cup light mayonnaise
- 1 tablespoon pickle relish
- 1 pound frozen bread dough, defrosted
- 1 egg, beaten
- sesame seeds
- vegetable or olive oil, in a spray bottle

Directions:

1. Combine the ground beef, steak seasoning and Worcestershire sauce in a large bowl. Divide the meat mixture into 12 equal portions. Cut the Cheddar cheese into twelve 2-inch squares, about ¼-inch thick. Stuff a square of cheese into the center of each portion of meat and shape into a 3-inch patty.
2. Make the slider sauce by combining the ketchup, mayonnaise, and relish in a small bowl. Set aside.
3. Cut the bread dough into twelve pieces. Shape each piece of dough into a ball and use a rolling pin to roll them out into 4-inch circles. Dollop ½ teaspoon of the slider sauce into the center of each dough circle. Place a beef patty on top of the sauce and wrap the dough around the patty, pinching the dough together to seal the pocket shut. Try not to stretch the dough too much when bringing the edges together. Brush both sides of the slider pocket with the beaten egg. Sprinkle sesame seeds on top of each pocket.
4. Preheat the air fryer to 350°F.
5. Spray or brush the bottom of the air fryer basket with oil. Air-fry the slider pockets four at a time. Transfer the slider pockets to the air fryer basket, seam side down and air-fry at 350°F for 10 minutes, until the dough is golden brown. Flip the slider pockets over and air-fry for another 3 minutes. When all the batches are done, pop all the sliders into the air fryer for a few minutes to re-heat and serve them hot out of the fryer.

Crabby Fries

Servings: 2

Cooking Time: 30 Minutes

Ingredients:

- 2 to 3 large russet potatoes, peeled and cut into ½-inch sticks
- 2 tablespoons vegetable oil
- 2 tablespoons butter
- 2 tablespoons flour
- 1 to 1½ cups milk
- ½ cup grated white Cheddar cheese
- pinch of nutmeg
- ½ teaspoon salt
- freshly ground black pepper
- 1 tablespoon Old Bay® Seasoning

Directions:

1. Bring a large saucepan of salted water to a boil on the stovetop while you peel and cut the potatoes. Blanch the potatoes in the boiling salted water for 4 minutes while you Preheat the air fryer to 400°F. Strain the potatoes and rinse them with cold water. Dry them well with a clean kitchen towel.
2. Toss the dried potato sticks gently with the oil and place them in the air fryer basket. Air-fry for 25 minutes, shaking the basket a few times while the fries cook to help them brown evenly.
3. While the fries are cooking, melt the butter in a medium saucepan. Whisk in the flour and cook for one minute. Slowly add 1 cup of milk, whisking constantly. Bring the mixture to a simmer and continue to whisk until it thickens. Remove the pan from the heat and stir in the Cheddar cheese. Add a pinch of nutmeg and season with salt and freshly ground black pepper. Transfer the warm cheese sauce to a serving dish. Thin with more milk if you want the sauce a little thinner.
4. As soon as the French fries have finished air-frying transfer them to a large bowl and season them with the Old Bay® Seasoning. Return the fries to the air fryer basket and air-fry for an additional 3 to 5 minutes. Serve immediately with the warm white Cheddar cheese sauce.

Apple Rollups

Servings: 8

Cooking Time: 5 Minutes

Ingredients:

- 8 slices whole wheat sandwich bread
- 4 ounces Colby Jack cheese, grated
- ½ small apple, chopped
- 2 tablespoons butter, melted

Directions:

1. Remove crusts from bread and flatten the slices with rolling pin. Don't be gentle. Press hard so that bread will be very thin.
2. Top bread slices with cheese and chopped apple, dividing the ingredients evenly.
3. Roll up each slice tightly and secure each with one or two toothpicks.
4. Brush outside of rolls with melted butter.
5. Place in air fryer basket and cook at 390°F for 5minutes, until outside is crisp and nicely browned.

Scotch Eggs

Servings: 6

Cooking Time: 12 Minutes

Ingredients:

- 7 Large eggs
- 1½ cups Corn flake crumbs (gluten-free, if a concern)
- 1½ pounds Bulk mild or hot breakfast sausage meat (gluten-free, if a concern)
- Vegetable oil spray
- For garnishing Coarse sea salt or kosher salt

Directions:

1. Bring a little more than 1 inch of water to a boil in a large saucepan set over high heat. Meanwhile, prepare a big bowl of ice water.
2. Set 4, 6, or 8 of the eggs in a vegetable steamer basket and lower them into the pot. Cover, reduce the heat to low, and steam for 10 minutes. Drain the eggs into a colander set in the sink, then put them in the ice water. Cool for 10 minutes, then peel the eggs. (Be careful: the whites are set but not the yolks!)
3. Preheat the air fryer to 375°F (or 380°F or 390°F, if one of these is the closest setting).
4. Lay a sheet of plastic wrap on a clean, dry work surface. Place ¼ pound (4 ounces) of the sausage meat in the center of the sheet, then press the sausage into an oval 7 inches long and about 5 inches wide at its widest part. Place a peeled egg in the center of the sausage, then carefully and gently (no awards for speed!) use the plastic wrap to fold the sausage up and around the egg. Remove the plastic wrap, dampen your clean hands, then smooth and seal the sausage over the egg. Repeat with the remaining sausage and eggs, using a fresh sheet of plastic wrap each time.
5. Set up and fill two shallow soup plates or small pie plates on your counter: one with the remaining egg(s) in it, well beaten until uniform, and the other with the corn flake crumbs. Roll the sausage-covered egg in the beaten egg. Let the excess slip back into the rest, then set the coated egg in the corn flake crumbs. Roll the egg in the corn flake crumbs to coat it evenly and well, even on the ends. Set aside, then coat the remaining sausage-covered eggs.
6. Give the crumbed eggs a generous coating of vegetable oil spray. Set them in the basket in one layer and air-fry undisturbed for 12 minutes, or until the coating is well browned. If the air fryer is at 390°F, the Scotch eggs may be done in 10 minutes.
7. Use kitchen tongs to transfer the eggs to a wire rack. Cool for at least 5 minutes or up to 30 minutes before serving. Split the eggs in half, sprinkle them with salt, and relish every bite.

Avocado Egg Rolls

Servings: 8

Cooking Time: 8 Minutes

Ingredients:

- 8 full-size egg roll wrappers
- 1 medium avocado, sliced into 8 pieces
- 1 cup cooked black beans, divided
- ½ cup mild salsa, divided
- ½ cup shredded Mexican cheese, divided
- ⅓ cup filtered water, divided
- ½ cup sour cream
- 1 teaspoon chipotle hot sauce

Directions:

1. Preheat the air fryer to 400°F.
2. Place the egg roll wrapper on a flat surface and place 1 strip of avocado down in the center.
3. Top the avocado with 2 tablespoons of black beans, 1 tablespoon of salsa, and 1 tablespoon of shredded cheese.
4. Place two of your fingers into the water, and then moisten the four outside edges of the egg roll wrapper with water (so the outer edges will secure shut).
5. Fold the bottom corner up, covering the filling. Then secure the sides over the top, remembering to lightly moisten them so they stick. Tightly roll the egg roll up and moisten the final flap of the wrapper and firmly press it into the egg roll to secure it shut.
6. Repeat Steps 2–5 until all 8 egg rolls are complete.
7. When ready to cook, spray the air fryer basket with olive oil spray and place the egg rolls into the basket. Depending on the size and type of air fryer you have, you may need to do this in two sets.
8. Cook for 4 minutes, flip, and then cook the remaining 4 minutes.
9. Repeat until all the egg rolls are cooked. Meanwhile, mix the sour cream with the hot sauce to serve as a dipping sauce.
10. Serve warm.

Sweet Chili Peanuts

Servings: 6

Cooking Time: 5 Minutes

Ingredients:

- 2 cups (10 ounces) Shelled raw peanuts
- 2 tablespoons Granulated white sugar
- 2 teaspoons Hot red pepper sauce, such as Cholula or Tabasco (gluten-free, if a concern)

Directions:

1. Preheat the air fryer to 400°F.
2. Toss the peanuts, sugar, and hot pepper sauce in a bowl until the peanuts are well coated.
3. When the machine is at temperature, pour the peanuts into the basket, spreading them into one layer as much as you can. Air-fry undisturbed for 3 minutes.
4. Shake the basket to rearrange the peanuts. Continue air-frying for 2 minutes more, shaking and stirring the peanuts every 30 seconds, until golden brown.
5. Pour the peanuts onto a large lipped baking sheet. Spread them into one layer and cool for 5 minutes before serving.

Meatball Arancini

Servings: 6

Cooking Time: 10 Minutes

Ingredients:

- 1⅓ cups Water
- ⅔ cup Raw white Arborio rice
- 2 teaspoons Butter
- ¼ teaspoon Table salt
- 2 Large egg(s), well beaten
- ¾ cup Seasoned Italian-style dried bread crumbs (gluten-free, if a concern)
- ⅓ cup (about 1 ounce) Finely grated Parmesan cheese
- 6 ½-ounce "bite-size" frozen meatballs (any variety, even vegan and/or gluten-free, if a concern), thawed
- Olive oil spray

Directions:

1. Combine the water, rice, butter, and salt in a small saucepan. Bring to a boil over medium-high heat, stirring occasionally. Cover, reduce the heat to very low, and simmer very slowly for 20 minutes.
2. Take the saucepan off the heat and let it stand, covered, for 10 minutes. Uncover it and fluff the rice. Cool for 20 minutes. (The rice can be made up to 1 hour in advance; keep it covered in its saucepan.)
3. Preheat the air fryer to 375°F .
4. Set up and fill two shallow soup plates or small bowls on your counter: one with the beaten egg(s) and one with the bread crumbs mixed with the grated cheese.
5. With clean but wet hands, scoop up about 3 tablespoons of the cooked rice and form it into a ball around a mini meatball, forming a sealed casing. Dip the ball in the egg(s) to coat completely, letting any excess egg slip back into the rest. Set the ball in the bread-crumb mixture and roll it gently to coat evenly but lightly all over. Set aside and continue making more rice balls.
6. Generously spray the balls with olive oil spray, then set them in the basket in one layer. They must not touch. Air-fry undisturbed for 10 minutes, or until crunchy and golden brown. Use kitchen tongs to gently transfer the balls to a wire rack. Cool for at least 5 minutes before serving.

Cauliflower "tater" Tots

Servings: 6

Cooking Time: 10 Minutes

Ingredients:

- 1 head of cauliflower
- 2 eggs
- ¼ cup all-purpose flour*
- ½ cup grated Parmesan cheese
- 1 teaspoon salt
- freshly ground black pepper
- vegetable or olive oil, in a spray bottle

Directions:

1. Grate the head of cauliflower with a box grater or finely chop it in a food processor. You should have about 3½ cups. Place the chopped cauliflower in the center of a clean kitchen towel and twist the towel tightly to squeeze all the water out of the cauliflower. (This can be done in two batches to make it easier to drain all the water from the cauliflower.)
2. Place the squeezed cauliflower in a large bowl. Add the eggs, flour, Parmesan cheese, salt and freshly ground black pepper. Shape the cauliflower into small cylinders or "tater tot" shapes, rolling roughly one tablespoon of the mixture at a time. Place the tots on a cookie sheet lined with paper towel to absorb any residual moisture. Spray the cauliflower tots all over with oil.
3. Preheat the air fryer to 400°F.
4. Air-fry the tots at 400°F, one layer at a time for 10 minutes, turning them over for the last few minutes of the cooking process for even browning. Season with salt and black pepper. Serve hot with your favorite dipping sauce.

Za'atar Garbanzo Beans

Servings: 6

Cooking Time: 12 Minutes

Ingredients:

- One 14.5-ounce can garbanzo beans, drained and rinsed
- 1 tablespoon extra-virgin olive oil
- 6 teaspoons za'atar seasoning mix
- 2 tablespoons chopped parsley
- Salt and pepper, to taste

Directions:

1. Preheat the air fryer to 390°F.
2. In a medium bowl, toss the garbanzo beans with olive oil and za'atar seasoning.
3. Pour the beans into the air fryer basket and cook for 12 minutes, or until toasted as you like. Stir every 3 minutes while roasting.
4. Remove the beans from the air fryer basket into a serving bowl, top with fresh chopped parsley, and season with salt and pepper.

Poultry Recipes

Spinach And Feta Stuffed Chicken Breasts

Servings: 4

Cooking Time: 27 Minutes

Ingredients:

- 1 (10-ounce) package frozen spinach, thawed and drained well
- 1 cup feta cheese, crumbled
- ½ teaspoon freshly ground black pepper
- 4 boneless chicken breasts
- salt and freshly ground black pepper
- 1 tablespoon olive oil

Directions:

1. Prepare the filling. Squeeze out as much liquid as possible from the thawed spinach. Rough chop the spinach and transfer it to a mixing bowl with the feta cheese and the freshly ground black pepper.
2. Prepare the chicken breast. Place the chicken breast on a cutting board and press down on the chicken breast with one hand to keep it stabilized. Make an incision about 1-inch long in the fattest side of the breast. Move the knife up and down inside the chicken breast, without poking through either the top or the bottom, or the other side of the breast. The inside pocket should be about 3-inches long, but the opening should only be about 1-inch wide. If this is too difficult, you can make the incision longer, but you will have to be more careful when cooking the chicken breast since this will expose more of the stuffing.
3. Once you have prepared the chicken breasts, use your fingers to stuff the filling into each pocket, spreading the mixture down as far as you can.
4. Preheat the air fryer to 380°F.
5. Lightly brush or spray the air fryer basket and the chicken breasts with olive oil. Transfer two of the stuffed chicken breasts to the air fryer. Air-fry for 12 minutes, turning the chicken breasts over halfway through the cooking time. Remove the chicken to a resting plate and air-fry the second two breasts for 12 minutes. Return the first batch of chicken to the air fryer with the second batch and air-fry for 3 more minutes. When the chicken is cooked, an instant read thermometer should register 165°F in the thickest part of the chicken, as well as in the stuffing.
6. Remove the chicken breasts and let them rest on a cutting board for 2 to 3 minutes. Slice the chicken on the bias and serve with the slices fanned out.

Thai Chicken Drumsticks

Servings: 4

Cooking Time: 20 Minutes

Ingredients:

- 2 tablespoons soy sauce
- ¼ cup rice wine vinegar
- 2 tablespoons chili garlic sauce
- 2 tablespoons sesame oil
- 1 teaspoon minced fresh ginger
- 2 teaspoons sugar
- ½ teaspoon ground coriander
- juice of 1 lime
- 8 chicken drumsticks (about 2½ pounds)
- ¼ cup chopped peanuts
- chopped fresh cilantro
- lime wedges

Directions:

1. Combine the soy sauce, rice wine vinegar, chili sauce, sesame oil, ginger, sugar, coriander and lime juice in a large bowl and mix together. Add the chicken drumsticks and marinate for 30 minutes.
2. Preheat the air fryer to 370°F.
3. Place the chicken in the air fryer basket. It's ok if the ends of the drumsticks overlap a little. Spoon half of the marinade over the chicken, and reserve the other half.
4. Air-fry for 10 minutes. Turn the chicken over and pour the rest of the marinade over the chicken. Air-fry for an additional 10 minutes.
5. Transfer the chicken to a plate to rest and cool to an edible temperature. Pour the marinade from the bottom of the air fryer into a small saucepan and bring it to a simmer over medium-high heat. Simmer the liquid for 2 minutes so that it thickens enough to coat the back of a spoon.
6. Transfer the chicken to a serving platter, pour the sauce over the chicken and sprinkle the chopped peanuts on top. Garnish with chopped cilantro and lime wedges.

Chicken Wellington

Servings: 2 Cooking Time: 31 Minutes

Ingredients:

- 2 (5-ounce) boneless, skinless chicken breasts
- ½ cup White Worcestershire sauce
- 3 tablespoons butter
- ½ cup finely diced onion (about ½ onion)
- 8 ounces button mushrooms, finely chopped
- ¼ cup chicken stock
- 2 tablespoons White Worcestershire sauce (or white wine)
- salt and freshly ground black pepper
- 1 tablespoon chopped fresh tarragon
- 2 sheets puff pastry, thawed
- 1 egg, beaten
- vegetable oil

Directions:

1. Place the chicken breasts in a shallow dish. Pour the White Worcestershire sauce over the chicken coating both sides and marinate for 30 minutes.
2. While the chicken is marinating, melt the butter in a large skillet over medium-high heat on the stovetop. Add the onion and sauté for a few minutes, until it starts to soften. Add the mushrooms and sauté for 5 minutes until the vegetables are brown and soft. Deglaze the skillet with the chicken stock, scraping up any bits from the bottom of the pan. Add the White Worcestershire sauce and simmer for 3 minutes until the mixture reduces and starts to thicken. Season with salt and freshly ground black pepper. Remove the mushroom mixture from the heat and stir in the fresh tarragon. Let the mushroom mixture cool.
3. Preheat the air fryer to 360°F.
4. Remove the chicken from the marinade and transfer it to the air fryer basket. Tuck the small end of the chicken breast under the thicker part to shape it into a circle rather than an oval. Pour the marinade over the chicken and air-fry for 10 minutes.
5. Roll out the puff pastry and cut out two 6-inch squares. Brush the perimeter of each square with the egg wash. Place half of the mushroom mixture in the center of each puff pastry square. Place the chicken breasts, top side down on the mushroom mixture. Starting with one corner of puff pastry and working in one direction, pull the pastry up over the chicken to enclose it and press the ends of the pastry together in the middle. Brush the pastry with the egg wash to seal the edges. Turn the Wellingtons over and set aside.
6. To make a decorative design with the remaining puff pastry, cut out four 10-inch strips. For each Wellington, twist two of the strips together, place them over the chicken breast wrapped in puff pastry,

and tuck the ends underneath to seal it. Brush the entire top and sides of the Wellingtons with the egg wash.

7. Preheat the air fryer to 350°F.
8. Spray or brush the air fryer basket with vegetable oil. Air-fry the chicken Wellingtons for 13 minutes. Carefully turn the Wellingtons over. Air-fry for another 8 minutes. Transfer to serving plates, light a candle and enjoy!

Thai Turkey And Zucchini Meatballs

Servings: 4

Cooking Time: 12 Minutes

Ingredients:

- 1½ cups grated zucchini,
- squeezed dry in a clean kitchen towel (about 1 large zucchini)
- 3 scallions, finely chopped
- 2 cloves garlic, minced
- 1 tablespoon grated fresh ginger
- 1 tablespoon finely chopped fresh cilantro
- zest of 1 lime
- 1 teaspoon salt
- freshly ground black pepper
- 1½ pounds ground turkey (a mix of light and dark meat)
- 2 eggs, lightly beaten
- 1 cup Thai sweet chili sauce (spring roll sauce)
- lime wedges, for serving

Directions:

1. Combine the zucchini, scallions, garlic, ginger, cilantro, lime zest, salt, pepper, ground turkey and eggs in a bowl and mix the ingredients together. Gently shape the mixture into 24 balls, about the size of golf balls.
2. Preheat the air fryer to 380°F.
3. Working in batches, air-fry the meatballs for 12 minutes, turning the meatballs over halfway through the cooking time. As soon as the meatballs have finished cooking, toss them in a bowl with the Thai sweet chili sauce to coat.
4. Serve the meatballs over rice noodles or white rice with the remaining Thai sweet chili sauce and lime wedges to squeeze over the top.

Chicken Nuggets

Servings: 20

Cooking Time: 14 Minutes Per Batch

Ingredients:

- 1 pound boneless, skinless chicken thighs, cut into 1-inch chunks
- ¾ teaspoon salt
- ½ teaspoon black pepper
- ½ teaspoon garlic powder
- ½ teaspoon onion powder
- ½ cup flour
- 2 eggs, beaten
- ½ cup panko breadcrumbs
- 3 tablespoons plain breadcrumbs
- oil for misting or cooking spray

Directions:

1. In the bowl of a food processor, combine chicken, ½ teaspoon salt, pepper, garlic powder, and onion powder. Process in short pulses until chicken is very finely chopped and well blended.
2. Place flour in one shallow dish and beaten eggs in another. In a third dish or plastic bag, mix together the panko crumbs, plain breadcrumbs, and ¼ teaspoon salt.
3. Shape chicken mixture into small nuggets. Dip nuggets in flour, then eggs, then panko crumb mixture.
4. Spray nuggets on both sides with oil or cooking spray and place in air fryer basket in a single layer, close but not overlapping.
5. Cook at 360°F for 10minutes. Spray with oil and cook 4 minutes, until chicken is done and coating is golden brown.
6. Repeat step 5 to cook remaining nuggets.

Southern-fried Chicken Livers

Servings: 4

Cooking Time: 12 Minutes

Ingredients:

- 2 eggs
- 2 tablespoons water
- ¾ cup flour
- 1½ cups panko breadcrumbs
- ½ cup plain breadcrumbs
- 1 teaspoon salt
- ½ teaspoon black pepper
- 20 ounces chicken livers, salted to taste
- oil for misting or cooking spray

Directions:

1. Beat together eggs and water in a shallow dish. Place the flour in a separate shallow dish.
2. In the bowl of a food processor, combine the panko, plain breadcrumbs, salt, and pepper. Process until well mixed and panko crumbs are finely crushed. Place crumbs in a third shallow dish.
3. Dip livers in flour, then egg wash, and then roll in panko mixture to coat well with crumbs.
4. Spray both sides of livers with oil or cooking spray. Cooking in two batches, place livers in air fryer basket in single layer.
5. Cook at 390°F for 7minutes. Spray livers, turn over, and spray again. Cook for 5 more minutes, until done inside and coating is golden brown.
6. Repeat to cook remaining livers.

Spicy Black Bean Turkey Burgers With Cumin-avocado Spread

Servings: 2

Cooking Time: 20 Minutes

Ingredients:

- 1 cup canned black beans, drained and rinsed
- ¾ pound lean ground turkey
- 2 tablespoons minced red onion
- 1 Jalapeño pepper, seeded and minced
- 2 tablespoons plain breadcrumbs
- ½ teaspoon chili powder
- ¼ teaspoon cayenne pepper
- salt, to taste
- olive or vegetable oil
- 2 slices pepper jack cheese
- toasted burger rolls, sliced tomatoes, lettuce leaves
- Cumin-Avocado Spread:
- 1 ripe avocado
- juice of 1 lime
- 1 teaspoon ground cumin
- ½ teaspoon salt
- 1 tablespoon chopped fresh cilantro
- freshly ground black pepper

Directions:

1. Place the black beans in a large bowl and smash them slightly with the back of a fork. Add the ground turkey, red onion, Jalapeño pepper, breadcrumbs, chili powder and cayenne pepper. Season with salt. Mix with your hands to combine all the ingredients and then shape them into 2 patties. Brush both sides of the burger patties with a little olive or vegetable oil.
2. Preheat the air fryer to 380°F.
3. Transfer the burgers to the air fryer basket and air-fry for 20 minutes, flipping them over halfway through the cooking process. Top the burgers with the pepper jack cheese (securing the slices to the burgers with a toothpick) for the last 2 minutes of the cooking process.
4. While the burgers are cooking, make the cumin avocado spread. Place the avocado, lime juice, cumin and salt in food processor and process until smooth. (For a chunkier spread, you can mash this by hand in a bowl.) Stir in the cilantro and season with freshly ground black pepper. Chill the spread until you are ready to serve.
5. When the burgers have finished cooking, remove them from the air fryer and let them rest on a plate, covered gently with aluminum foil. Brush a little olive oil on the insides of the burger rolls. Place the rolls, cut side up, into the air fryer basket and air-fry at 400°F for 1 minute to toast and warm them.
6. Spread the cumin-avocado spread on the rolls and build your burgers with lettuce and sliced tomatoes and any other ingredient you like. Serve warm with a side of sweet potato fries.

Coconut Chicken With Apricot-ginger Sauce

Servings: 4

Cooking Time: 8 Minutes Per Batch

Ingredients:

- 1½ pounds boneless, skinless chicken tenders, cut in large chunks (about 1¼ inches)
- salt and pepper
- ½ cup cornstarch
- 2 eggs
- 1 tablespoon milk
- 3 cups shredded coconut (see below)
- oil for misting or cooking spray
- Apricot-Ginger Sauce
- ½ cup apricot preserves
- 2 tablespoons white vinegar
- ¼ teaspoon ground ginger
- ¼ teaspoon low-sodium soy sauce
- 2 teaspoons white or yellow onion, grated or finely minced

Directions:

1. Mix all ingredients for the Apricot-Ginger Sauce well and let sit for flavors to blend while you cook the chicken.
2. Season chicken chunks with salt and pepper to taste.
3. Place cornstarch in a shallow dish.
4. In another shallow dish, beat together eggs and milk.
5. Place coconut in a third shallow dish. (If also using panko breadcrumbs, as suggested below, stir them to mix well.)
6. Spray air fryer basket with oil or cooking spray.
7. Dip each chicken chunk into cornstarch, shake off excess, and dip in egg mixture.
8. Shake off excess egg mixture and roll lightly in coconut or coconut mixture. Spray with oil.
9. Place coated chicken chunks in air fryer basket in a single layer, close together but without sides touching.
10. Cook at 360°F for 4minutes, stop, and turn chunks over.
11. Cook an additional 4 minutes or until chicken is done inside and coating is crispy brown.
12. Repeat steps 9 through 11 to cook remaining chicken chunks.

Cornish Hens With Honey-lime Glaze

Servings: 2

Cooking Time: 30 Minutes

Ingredients:

- 1 Cornish game hen (1½–2 pounds)
- 1 tablespoon honey
- 1 tablespoon lime juice
- 1 teaspoon poultry seasoning
- salt and pepper
- cooking spray

Directions:

1. To split the hen into halves, cut through breast bone and down one side of the backbone.
2. Mix the honey, lime juice, and poultry seasoning together and brush or rub onto all sides of the hen. Season to taste with salt and pepper.
3. Spray air fryer basket with cooking spray and place hen halves in the basket, skin-side down.
4. Cook at 330°F for 30 minutes. Hen will be done when juices run clear when pierced at leg joint with a fork. Let hen rest for 5 to 10minutes before cutting.

Taquitos

Servings: 12

Cooking Time: 6 Minutes Per Batch

Ingredients:

- 1 teaspoon butter
- 2 tablespoons chopped green onions
- 1 cup cooked chicken, shredded
- 2 tablespoons chopped green chiles
- 2 ounces Pepper Jack cheese, shredded
- 4 tablespoons salsa
- ½ teaspoon lime juice
- ¼ teaspoon cumin
- ½ teaspoon chile powder
- ⅛ teaspoon garlic powder
- 12 corn tortillas
- oil for misting or cooking spray

Directions:

1. Melt butter in a saucepan over medium heat. Add green onions and sauté a minute or two, until tender.
2. Remove from heat and stir in the chicken, green chiles, cheese, salsa, lime juice, and seasonings.
3. Preheat air fryer to 390°F.
4. To soften refrigerated tortillas, wrap in damp paper towels and microwave for 30 to 60 seconds, until slightly warmed.
5. Remove one tortilla at a time, keeping others covered with the damp paper towels. Place a heaping tablespoon of filling into tortilla, roll up and secure with toothpick. Spray all sides with oil or cooking spray.
6. Place taquitos in air fryer basket, either in a single layer or stacked. To stack, leave plenty of space between taquitos and alternate the direction of the layers, 4 on the bottom lengthwise, then 4 more on top crosswise.
7. Cook for 6minutes or until brown and crispy.
8. Repeat steps 6 and 7 to cook remaining taquitos.
9. Serve hot with guacamole, sour cream, salsa or all three!

Beef， Pork & Lamb Recipes

Pepper Steak

Servings: 4

Cooking Time: 30 Minutes

Ingredients:

- 2 tablespoons cornstarch
- 1 tablespoon sugar
- ¾ cup beef broth
- ¼ cup hoisin sauce
- 3 tablespoons soy sauce
- 1 teaspoon sesame oil
- ½ teaspoon freshly ground black pepper
- 1½ pounds boneless New York strip steaks, sliced into ½-inch strips
- 1 onion, sliced
- 3 small bell peppers, red, yellow and green, sliced

Directions:

1. Whisk the cornstarch and sugar together in a large bowl to break up any lumps in the cornstarch. Add the beef broth and whisk until combined and smooth. Stir in the hoisin sauce, soy sauce, sesame oil and freshly ground black pepper. Add the beef, onion and peppers, and toss to coat. Marinate the beef and vegetables at room temperature for 30 minutes, stirring a few times to keep meat and vegetables coated.
2. Preheat the air fryer to 350°F.
3. Transfer the beef, onion, and peppers to the air fryer basket with tongs, reserving the marinade. Air-fry the beef and vegetables for 30 minutes, stirring well two or three times during the cooking process.
4. While the beef is air-frying, bring the reserved marinade to a simmer in a small saucepan over medium heat on the stovetop. Simmer for 5 minutes until the sauce thickens.
5. When the steak and vegetables have finished cooking, transfer them to a serving platter. Pour the hot sauce over the pepper steak and serve with white rice.

Vietnamese Beef Lettuce Wraps

Servings: 4

Cooking Time: 12 Minutes

Ingredients:

- ⅓ cup low-sodium soy sauce*
- 2 teaspoons fish sauce*
- 2 teaspoons brown sugar
- 1 tablespoon chili paste
- juice of 1 lime
- 2 cloves garlic, minced
- 2 teaspoons fresh ginger, minced
- 1 pound beef sirloin
- Sauce
- ⅓ cup low-sodium soy sauce*
- juice of 2 limes
- 1 tablespoon mirin wine
- 2 teaspoons chili paste
- Serving
- 1 head butter lettuce
- ½ cup julienned carrots
- ½ cup julienned cucumber
- ½ cup sliced radishes, sliced into half moons
- 2 cups cooked rice noodles
- ⅓ cup chopped peanuts

Directions:

1. Combine the soy sauce, fish sauce, brown sugar, chili paste, lime juice, garlic and ginger in a bowl. Slice the beef into thin slices, then cut those slices in half. Add the beef to the marinade and marinate for 1 to 3 hours in the refrigerator. When you are ready to cook, remove the steak from the refrigerator and let it sit at room temperature for 30 minutes.
2. Preheat the air fryer to 400°F.
3. Transfer the beef and marinade to the air fryer basket. Air-fry at 400°F for 12 minutes, shaking the basket a few times during the cooking process.
4. While the beef is cooking, prepare a wrap-building station. Combine the soy sauce, lime juice, mirin wine and chili paste in a bowl and transfer to a little pouring vessel. Separate the lettuce leaves from the head of lettuce and put them in a serving bowl. Place the carrots, cucumber, radish, rice noodles and chopped peanuts all in separate serving bowls.
5. When the beef has finished cooking, transfer it to another serving bowl and invite your guests to build their wraps. To build the wraps, place some beef in a lettuce leaf and top with carrots, cucumbers, some rice noodles and chopped peanuts. Drizzle a little sauce over top, fold the lettuce around the ingredients and enjoy!

Pork & Beef Egg Rolls

Servings: 8

Cooking Time: 8 Minutes

Ingredients:

- ¼ pound very lean ground beef
- ¼ pound lean ground pork
- 1 tablespoon soy sauce
- 1 teaspoon olive oil
- ½ cup grated carrots
- 2 green onions, chopped
- 2 cups grated Napa cabbage
- ¼ cup chopped water chestnuts
- ¼ teaspoon salt
- ¼ teaspoon garlic powder
- ¼ teaspoon black pepper
- 1 egg
- 1 tablespoon water
- 8 egg roll wraps
- oil for misting or cooking spray

Directions:

1. In a large skillet, brown beef and pork with soy sauce. Remove cooked meat from skillet, drain, and set aside.
2. Pour off any excess grease from skillet. Add olive oil, carrots, and onions. Sauté until barely tender, about 1 minute.
3. Stir in cabbage, cover, and cook for 1 minute or just until cabbage slightly wilts. Remove from heat.
4. In a large bowl, combine the cooked meats and vegetables, water chestnuts, salt, garlic powder, and pepper. Stir well. If needed, add more salt to taste.
5. Beat together egg and water in a small bowl.
6. Fill egg roll wrappers, using about ¼ cup of filling for each wrap. Roll up and brush all over with egg wash to seal. Spray very lightly with olive oil or cooking spray.
7. Place 4 egg rolls in air fryer basket and cook at 390°F for 4minutes. Turn over and cook 4 more minutes, until golden brown and crispy.
8. Repeat to cook remaining egg rolls.

Chicken-fried Steak

Servings: 2

Cooking Time: 12 Minutes

Ingredients:

- 1½ cups All-purpose flour
- 2 Large egg(s)
- 2 tablespoons Regular or low-fat sour cream
- 2 tablespoons Worcestershire sauce
- 2 ¼-pound thin beef cube steak(s)
- Vegetable oil spray

Directions:

1. Preheat the air fryer to 400°F.
2. Set up and fill two shallow soup plates or small pie plates on your counter: one for the flour; and one for the egg(s), whisked with the sour cream and Worcestershire sauce until uniform.
3. Dredge a piece of beef in the flour, coating it well on both sides and even along the edge. Shake off any excess; then dip the meat in the egg mixture, coating both sides while retaining the flour on the meat. Let any excess egg mixture slip back into the rest. Dredge the meat in the flour once again, coating all surfaces well. Gently shake off the excess coating and set the steak aside if you're coating another steak or two. Once done, coat the steak(s) on both sides with the vegetable oil spray.
4. Set the steak(s) in the basket. If there's more than one steak, make sure they do not overlap or even touch, although the smallest gap between them is enough to get them crunchy. Air-fry undisturbed for 6 minutes.
5. Use kitchen tongs to pick up one of the steaks. Coat it again on both sides with vegetable oil spray. Turn it upside down and set it back in the basket with that same regard for the space between them in larger batches. Repeat with any other steaks. Continue air-frying undisturbed for 6 minutes, or until golden brown and crunchy.
6. Use kitchen tongs to transfer the steak(s) to a wire rack. Cool for 5 minutes before serving.

Barbecue-style Beef Cube Steak

Servings: 2

Cooking Time: 14 Minutes

Ingredients:

- 2 4-ounce beef cube steak(s)
- 2 cups (about 8 ounces) Fritos (original flavor) or a generic corn chip equivalent, crushed to crumbs (see here)
- 6 tablespoons Purchased smooth barbecue sauce, any flavor (gluten-free, if a concern)

Directions:

1. Preheat the air fryer to 375°F .
2. Spread the Fritos crumbs in a shallow soup plate or a small pie plate. Rub the barbecue sauce onto both sides of the steak(s). Dredge the steak(s) in the Fritos crumbs to coat well and thoroughly, turning several times and pressing down to get the little bits to adhere to the meat.
3. When the machine is at temperature, set the steak(s) in the basket. Leave as much air space between them as possible if you're working with more than one piece of beef. Air-fry undisturbed for 12 minutes, or until lightly brown and crunchy. If the machine is at 360°F, you may need to add 2 minutes to the cooking time.
4. Use kitchen tongs to transfer the steak(s) to a wire rack. Cool for 5 minutes before serving.

Venison Backstrap

Servings: 4

Cooking Time: 10 Minutes

Ingredients:

- 2 eggs
- ¼ cup milk
- 1 cup whole wheat flour
- ½ teaspoon salt
- ¼ teaspoon pepper
- 1 pound venison backstrap, sliced
- salt and pepper
- oil for misting or cooking spray

Directions:

1. Beat together eggs and milk in a shallow dish.
2. In another shallow dish, combine the flour, salt, and pepper. Stir to mix well.
3. Sprinkle venison steaks with additional salt and pepper to taste. Dip in flour, egg wash, then in flour again, pressing in coating.
4. Spray steaks with oil or cooking spray on both sides.
5. Cooking in 2 batches, place steaks in the air fryer basket in a single layer. Cook at 360°F for 8minutes. Spray with oil, turn over, and spray other side. Cook for 2 minutes longer, until coating is crispy brown and meat is done to your liking.
6. Repeat to cook remaining venison.

Italian Meatballs

Servings: 4

Cooking Time: 12 Minutes

Ingredients:

- 12 ounces lean ground beef
- 4 ounces Italian sausage, casing removed
- ½ cup breadcrumbs
- 1 cup grated Parmesan cheese
- 1 egg
- 2 tablespoons milk
- 2 teaspoons Italian seasoning
- ½ teaspoon onion powder
- ½ teaspoon garlic powder
- Pinch of red pepper flakes

Directions:

1. In a large bowl, place all the ingredients and mix well. Roll out 24 meatballs.
2. Preheat the air fryer to 360°F.
3. Place the meatballs in the air fryer basket and cook for 12 minutes, tossing every 4 minutes. Using a food thermometer, check to ensure the internal temperature of the meatballs is 165°F.

City “chicken”

Servings: 3

Cooking Time: 10 Minutes

Ingredients:

- 1 pound Pork tenderloin, cut into 2-inch cubes
- ½ cup All-purpose flour or tapioca flour
- 1 Large egg(s)
- 1 teaspoon Dried poultry seasoning blend
- 1¼ cups Plain panko bread crumbs (gluten-free, if a concern)
- Vegetable oil spray

Directions:

1. Preheat the air fryer to 350°F .
2. Thread 3 or 4 pieces of pork on a 4-inch bamboo skewer. You’ll need 2 or 3 skewers for a small batch, 3 or 4 for a medium, and up to 6 for a large batch.
3. Set up and fill three shallow soup plates or small pie plates on your counter: one for the flour; one for the egg(s), beaten with the poultry seasoning until foamy; and one for the bread crumbs.
4. Dip and roll one skewer into the flour, coating all sides of the meat. Gently shake off any excess flour, then dip and roll the skewer in the egg mixture. Let any excess egg mixture slip back into the rest, then set the skewer in the bread crumbs and roll it around, pressing gently, until the exterior surfaces of the meat are evenly coated. Generously coat the meat on the skewer with vegetable oil spray. Set aside and continue dredging, dipping, coating, and spraying the remaining skewers.
5. Set the skewers in the basket in one layer and air-fry undisturbed for 10 minutes, or until brown and crunchy.
6. Use kitchen tongs to transfer the skewers to a wire rack. Cool for a minute or two before serving.

Crispy Lamb Shoulder Chops

Servings: 3

Cooking Time: 28 Minutes

Ingredients:

- ¾ cup All-purpose flour or gluten-free all-purpose flour
- 2 teaspoons Mild paprika
- 2 teaspoons Table salt
- 1½ teaspoons Garlic powder
- 1½ teaspoons Dried sage leaves
- 3 6-ounce bone-in lamb shoulder chops, any excess fat trimmed
- Olive oil spray

Directions:

1. Whisk the flour, paprika, salt, garlic powder, and sage in a large bowl until the mixture is of a uniform color. Add the chops and toss well to coat. Transfer them to a cutting board.
2. Preheat the air fryer to 375°F .
3. When the machine is at temperature, again dredge the chops one by one in the flour mixture. Lightly coat both sides of each chop with olive oil spray before putting it in the basket. Continue on with the remaining chop(s), leaving air space between them in the basket.
4. Air-fry, turning once, for 25 minutes, or until the chops are well browned and tender when pierced with the point of a paring knife. If the machine is at 360°F, you may need to add up to 3 minutes to the cooking time.
5. Use kitchen tongs to transfer the chops to a wire rack. Cool for 5 minutes before serving.

Fried Spam

Servings: 2

Cooking Time: 12 Minutes

Ingredients:

- ½ cup All-purpose flour or gluten-free all-purpose flour
- 1 Large egg(s)
- 1 tablespoon Wasabi paste
- 1⅓ cups Plain panko bread crumbs (gluten-free, if a concern)
- 4 ½-inch-thick Spam slices
- Vegetable oil spray

Directions:

1. Preheat the air fryer to 400°F.
2. Set up and fill three shallow soup plates or small pie plates on your counter: one for the flour; one for the egg(s), whisked with the wasabi paste until uniform; and one for the bread crumbs.
3. Dip a slice of Spam in the flour, coating both sides. Slip it into the egg mixture and turn to coat on both sides, even along the edges. Let any excess egg mixture slip back into the rest, then set the slice in the bread crumbs. Turn it several times, pressing gently to make an even coating on both sides. Generously coat both sides of the slice with vegetable oil spray. Set aside so you can dip, coat, and spray the remaining slice(s).
4. Set the slices in the basket in a single layer so that they don't touch (even if they're close together). Air-fry undisturbed for 12 minutes, or until very brown and quite crunchy.
5. Use kitchen tongs to transfer the slices to a wire rack. Cool for a minute or two before serving.

Vegetable Side Dishes Recipes

Roman Artichokes

Servings: 4

Cooking Time: 12 Minutes

Ingredients:

- 2 9-ounce box(es) frozen artichoke heart quarters, thawed
- 1½ tablespoons Olive oil
- 2 teaspoons Minced garlic
- 1 teaspoon Table salt
- Up to ½ teaspoon Red pepper flakes

Directions:

1. Preheat the air fryer to 400°F.
2. Gently toss the artichoke heart quarters, oil, garlic, salt, and red pepper flakes in a bowl until the quarters are well coated.
3. When the machine is at temperature, scrape the contents of the bowl into the basket. Spread the artichoke heart quarters out into as close to one layer as possible. Air-fry undisturbed for 8 minutes. Gently toss and rearrange the quarters so that any covered or touching parts are now exposed to the air currents, then air-fry undisturbed for 4 minutes more, until very crisp.
4. Gently pour the contents of the basket onto a wire rack. Cool for a few minutes before serving.

Crispy Cauliflower Puffs

Servings: 12

Cooking Time: 9 Minutes

Ingredients:

- 1½ cups Riced cauliflower
- 1 cup (about 4 ounces) Shredded Monterey Jack cheese
- ¾ cup Seasoned Italian-style panko bread crumbs (gluten-free, if a concern)
- 2 tablespoons plus 1 teaspoon All-purpose flour or potato starch
- 2 tablespoons plus 1 teaspoon Vegetable oil
- 1 plus 1 large yolk Large egg(s)
- ¾ teaspoon Table salt
- Vegetable oil spray

Directions:

1. Preheat the air fryer to 375°F .
2. Stir the riced cauliflower, cheese, bread crumbs, flour or potato starch, oil, egg(s) and egg yolk (if necessary), and salt in a large bowl to make a thick batter.
3. Using 2 tablespoons of the batter, form a compact ball between your clean, dry palms. Set it aside and continue forming more balls: 7 more for a small batch, 11 more for a medium batch, or 15 more for a large batch.
4. Generously coat the balls on all sides with vegetable oil spray. Set them in the basket with as much air space between them as possible. Air-fry undisturbed for 7 minutes, or until golden brown and crisp. If the machine is at 360°F, you may need to add 2 minutes to the cooking time.
5. Gently pour the contents of the basket onto a wire rack. Cool the puffs for 5 minutes before serving.

Buttermilk Biscuits

Servings: 5

Cooking Time: 14 Minutes

Ingredients:

- 1⅔ cups, plus more for dusting All-purpose flour
- 1½ teaspoons Baking powder
- ¼ teaspoon Table salt
- 3 tablespoons plus 1 teaspoon Butter, cold and cut into small pieces
- ½ cup plus ½ tablespoon Cold buttermilk, regular or low-fat
- 2½ tablespoons Butter, melted and cooled

Directions:

1. Preheat the air fryer to 400°F.
2. Mix the flour, baking powder, and salt in a large bowl. Use a pastry cutter or a sturdy flatware fork to cut the cold butter pieces into the flour mixture, working the fat through the tines again and again until the mixture resembles coarse dry sand. Stir in the buttermilk to make a dough.
3. Very lightly dust a clean, dry work surface with flour. Turn the dough out onto it, dip your clean hands into flour, and press the dough into a ¾-inch-thick circle. Use a 3-inch round cookie cutter or sturdy drinking glass to cut the dough into rounds. Gather the dough scraps together, lightly shape again into a ¾-inch-thick circle, and cut out a few more rounds. You'll end up with 4 raw biscuits for a small air fryer, 5 for a medium, or 6 for a large.
4. For a small air fryer, brush the inside of a 6-inch round cake pan with a little more than half of the melted butter, then set the 4 raw biscuits in it, letting them touch but without squishing them.
5. For a medium air fryer, do the same with half of the melted butter in a 7-inch round cake pan and 5 raw biscuits.
6. And for a large air fryer, use a little more than half the melted butter to brush the inside of an 8-inch round cake pan, and set the 6 raw biscuits in it in the same way.
7. Brush the tops of the raw biscuits with the remaining melted butter.
8. Air-fry undisturbed for 14 minutes, or until the biscuits are golden brown and dry to the touch.
9. Using kitchen tongs and a nonstick-safe spatula, two hot pads, or silicone baking mitts, remove the cake pan from the basket and set it on a wire rack. Cool undisturbed for a couple of minutes. Turn the biscuits out onto the wire rack to cool for a couple of minutes more before serving.

Zucchini Boats With Ham And Cheese

Servings: 4

Cooking Time: 12 Minutes

Ingredients:

- 2 6-inch-long zucchini
- 2 ounces Thinly sliced deli ham, any rind removed, meat roughly chopped
- 4 Dry-packed sun-dried tomatoes, chopped
- ⅓ cup Purchased pesto
- ¼ cup Packaged mini croutons
- ¼ cup (about 1 ounce) Shredded semi-firm mozzarella cheese

Directions:

1. Preheat the air fryer to 375°F .
2. Split the zucchini in half lengthwise and use a flatware spoon or a serrated grapefruit spoon to scoop out the insides of the halves, leaving at least a ¼-inch border all around the zucchini half. (You can save the scooped out insides to add to soups and stews—or even freeze it for a much later use.)
3. Mix the ham, sun-dried tomatoes, pesto, croutons, and half the cheese in a bowl until well combined. Pack this mixture into the zucchini "shells." Top them with the remaining cheese.
4. Set them stuffing side up in the basket without touching (even a fraction of an inch between them is enough room). Air-fry undisturbed for 12 minutes, or until softened and browned, with the cheese melted on top.
5. Use a nonstick-safe spatula to transfer the zucchini boats stuffing side up on a wire rack. Cool for 5 or 10 minutes before serving.

Buttery Rolls

Servings: 6

Cooking Time: 14 Minutes

Ingredients:

- 6½ tablespoons Room-temperature whole or low-fat milk
- 3 tablespoons plus 1 teaspoon Butter, melted and cooled
- 3 tablespoons plus 1 teaspoon (or 1 medium egg, well beaten) Pasteurized egg substitute, such as Egg Beaters
- 1½ tablespoons Granulated white sugar
- 1¼ teaspoons Instant yeast
- ¼ teaspoon Table salt
- 2 cups, plus more for dusting All-purpose flour
- Vegetable oil
- Additional melted butter, for brushing

Directions:

1. Stir the milk, melted butter, pasteurized egg substitute (or whole egg), sugar, yeast, and salt in a medium bowl to combine. Stir in the flour just until the mixture makes a soft dough.
2. Lightly flour a clean, dry work surface. Turn the dough out onto the work surface. Knead the dough for 5 minutes to develop the gluten.
3. Lightly oil the inside of a clean medium bowl. Gather the dough into a compact ball and set it in the bowl. Turn the dough over so that its surface has oil on it all over. Cover the bowl tightly with plastic wrap and set aside in a warm, draft-free place until the dough has doubled in bulk, about 1½ hours.
4. Punch down the dough, then turn it out onto a clean, dry work surface. Divide it into 5 even balls for a small batch, 6 balls for a medium batch, or 8 balls for a large one.
5. For a small batch, lightly oil the inside of a 6-inch round cake pan and set the balls around its perimeter, separating them as much as possible.
6. For a medium batch, lightly oil the inside of a 7-inch round cake pan and set the balls in it with one ball at its center, separating them as much as possible.
7. For a large batch, lightly oil the inside of an 8-inch round cake pan and set the balls in it with one at the center, separating them as much as possible.
8. Cover with plastic wrap and set aside to rise for 30 minutes.
9. Preheat the air fryer to 350°F .
10. Uncover the pan and brush the rolls with a little melted butter, perhaps ½ teaspoon per roll. When the machine is at temperature, set the cake pan in the basket. Air-fry undisturbed for 14 minutes, or until the rolls have risen and browned.

11. Using kitchen tongs and a nonstick-safe spatula, two hot pads, or silicone baking mitts, transfer the cake pan from the basket to a wire rack. Cool the rolls in the pan for a minute or two. Turn the rolls out onto a wire rack, set them top side up again, and cool for at least another couple of minutes before serving warm.

Acorn Squash Halves With Maple Butter Glaze

Servings: 2

Cooking Time: 33 Minutes

Ingredients:

- 1 medium (1 to 1¼ pounds) Acorn squash
- Vegetable oil spray
- ¼ teaspoon Table salt
- 1½ tablespoons Butter, melted
- 1½ tablespoons Maple syrup

Directions:

1. Preheat the air fryer to 325°F (or 330°F, if that's the closest setting).
2. Cut a squash in half through the stem end. Use a flatware spoon (preferably, a serrated grapefruit spoon) to scrape out and discard the seeds and membranes in each half. Use a paring knife to make a crisscross pattern of cuts about ½ inch apart and ¼ inch deep across the "meat" of the squash. If working with a second squash, repeat this step for that one.
3. Generously coat the cut side of the squash halves with vegetable oil spray. Sprinkle the halves with the salt. Set them in the basket cut side up with at least ¼ inch between them. Air-fry undisturbed for 30 minutes.
4. Increase the machine's temperature to 400°F. Mix the melted butter and syrup in a small bowl until uniform. Brush this mixture over the cut sides of the squash(es), letting it pool in the center. Air-fry undisturbed for 3 minutes, or until the glaze is bubbling.
5. Use a nonstick-safe spatula and kitchen tongs to transfer the squash halves cut side up to a wire rack. Cool for 5 to 10 minutes before serving.

Summer Vegetables With Balsamic Drizzle, Goat Cheese And Basil

Servings: 2

Cooking Time: 17 Minutes

Ingredients:

- 1 cup balsamic vinegar
- 1 zucchini, sliced
- 1 yellow squash, sliced
- 2 tablespoons olive oil
- 1 clove garlic, minced
- ½ teaspoon Italian seasoning
- salt and freshly ground black pepper
- ½ cup cherry tomatoes, halved
- 2 ounces crumbled goat cheese
- 2 tablespoons chopped fresh basil, plus more leaves for garnish

Directions:

1. Place the balsamic vinegar in a small saucepot on the stovetop. Bring the vinegar to a boil, lower the heat and simmer uncovered for 20 minutes, until the mixture reduces and thickens. Set aside to cool.
2. Preheat the air fryer to 390°F.
3. Combine the zucchini and yellow squash in a large bowl. Add the olive oil, minced garlic, Italian seasoning, salt and pepper and toss to coat.
4. Air-fry the vegetables at 390°F for 10 minutes, shaking the basket several times during the cooking process. Add the cherry tomatoes and continue to air-fry for another 5 minutes. Sprinkle the goat cheese over the vegetables and air-fry for 2 more minutes.
5. Transfer the vegetables to a serving dish, drizzle with the balsamic reduction and season with freshly ground black pepper. Garnish with the fresh basil leaves.

Glazed Carrots

Servings: 4

Cooking Time: 10 Minutes

Ingredients:

- 2 teaspoons honey
- 1 teaspoon orange juice
- ½ teaspoon grated orange rind
- ⅛ teaspoon ginger
- 1 pound baby carrots
- 2 teaspoons olive oil
- ¼ teaspoon salt

Directions:

1. Combine honey, orange juice, grated rind, and ginger in a small bowl and set aside.
2. Toss the carrots, oil, and salt together to coat well and pour them into the air fryer basket.
3. Cook at 390°F for 5minutes. Shake basket to stir a little and cook for 4 minutes more, until carrots are barely tender.
4. Pour carrots into air fryer baking pan.
5. Stir the honey mixture to combine well, pour glaze over carrots, and stir to coat.
6. Cook at 360°F for 1 minute or just until heated through.

Tuna Platter

Servings: 4

Cooking Time: 9 Minutes

Ingredients:

- 4 new potatoes, boiled in their jackets
- ½ cup vinaigrette dressing, plus 2 tablespoons
- ½ pound fresh green beans, cut in half-inch pieces and steamed
- 1 tablespoon Herbes de Provence
- 1 tablespoon minced shallots
- 1½ tablespoons tarragon vinegar
- 4 tuna steaks, each ¾-inch thick, about 1 pound
- salt and pepper
- Salad
- 8 cups chopped romaine lettuce
- 12 grape tomatoes, halved lengthwise
- ½ cup pitted olives (black, green, nicoise, or combination)
- 2 boiled eggs, peeled and halved lengthwise

Directions:

1. Quarter potatoes and toss with 1 tablespoon salad dressing.
2. Toss the warm beans with the other tablespoon of salad dressing. Set both aside while you prepare the tuna.
3. Mix together the herbs, shallots, and vinegar and rub into all sides of tuna. Season fish to taste with salt and pepper.
4. Cook tuna at 390°F for 7minutes and check. If needed, cook 2 minutes longer, until tuna is barely pink in the center.
5. Spread the lettuce over a large platter.
6. Slice the tuna steaks in ½-inch pieces and arrange them in the center of the lettuce.
7. Place the remaining ingredients around the tuna. Diners create their own plates by selecting what they want from the platter. Pass remainder of salad dressing at the table.

Roasted Broccoli And Red Bean Salad

Servings: 3

Cooking Time: 14 Minutes

Ingredients:

- 3 cups (about 1 pound) 1- to 1½-inch fresh broccoli florets (not frozen)
- 1½ tablespoons Olive oil spray
- 1¼ cups Canned red kidney beans, drained and rinsed
- 3 tablespoons Minced yellow or white onion
- 2 tablespoons plus 1 teaspoon Red wine vinegar
- ¾ teaspoon Dried oregano
- ¼ teaspoon Table salt
- ¼ teaspoon Ground black pepper

Directions:

1. Preheat the air fryer to 375°F .
2. Put the broccoli florets in a big bowl, coat them generously with olive oil spray, then toss to coat all surfaces, even down into the crannies, spraying them a couple of times more.
3. Pour the florets into the basket, spreading them into as close to one layer as you can. Air-fry for 12 minutes, tossing and rearranging the florets twice so that any touching or covered parts are eventually exposed to the air currents, until light browned but still a bit firm. (If the machine is at 360°F, you may need to add 2 minutes to the cooking time.)
4. Dump the contents of the basket onto a large cutting board. Cool for a minute or two, then chop the florets into small bits. Scrape these into a bowl and add the kidney beans, onion, vinegar, oregano, salt, and pepper. Toss well and serve warm or at room temperature.

Desserts And Sweets

Hasselback Apple Crisp

Servings: 4

Cooking Time: 20 Minutes

Ingredients:

- 2 large Gala apples, peeled, cored and cut in half
- ¼ cup butter, melted
- ½ teaspoon ground cinnamon
- 2 tablespoons sugar
- Topping
- 3 tablespoons butter, melted
- 2 tablespoons brown sugar
- ¼ cup chopped pecans
- 2 tablespoons rolled oats*
- 1 tablespoon flour*
- vanilla ice cream
- caramel sauce

Directions:

1. Place the apples cut side down on a cutting board. Slicing from stem end to blossom end, make 8 to 10 slits down the apple halves but only slice three quarters of the way through the apple, not all the way through to the cutting board.
2. Preheat the air fryer to 330°F and pour a little water into the bottom of the air fryer drawer. (This will help prevent the grease that drips into the bottom drawer from burning and smoking.)
3. Transfer the apples to the air fryer basket, flat side down. Combine ¼ cup of melted butter, cinnamon and sugar in a small bowl. Brush this butter mixture onto the apples and air-fry at 330°F for 15 minutes. Baste the apples several times with the butter mixture during the cooking process.
4. While the apples are air-frying, make the filling. Combine 3 tablespoons of melted butter with the brown sugar, pecans, rolled oats and flour in a bowl. Stir with a fork until the mixture resembles small crumbles.
5. When the timer on the air fryer is up, spoon the topping down the center of the apples. Air-fry at 330°F for an additional 5 minutes.
6. Transfer the apples to a serving plate and serve with vanilla ice cream and caramel sauce.

Dark Chocolate Peanut Butter S'mores

Servings: 4

Cooking Time: 6 Minutes

Ingredients:

- 4 graham cracker sheets
- 4 marshmallows
- 4 teaspoons chunky peanut butter
- 4 ounces dark chocolate
- ½ teaspoon ground cinnamon

Directions:

1. Preheat the air fryer to 390°F. Break the graham crackers in half so you have 8 pieces.
2. Place 4 pieces of graham cracker on the bottom of the air fryer. Top each with one of the marshmallows and bake for 6 or 7 minutes, or until the marshmallows have a golden brown center.
3. While cooking, slather each of the remaining graham crackers with 1 teaspoon peanut butter.
4. When baking completes, carefully remove each of the graham crackers, add 1 ounce of dark chocolate on top of the marshmallow, and lightly sprinkle with cinnamon. Top with the remaining peanut butter graham cracker to make the sandwich. Serve immediately.

Wild Blueberry Sweet Empanadas

Servings: 12

Cooking Time: 8 Minutes

Ingredients:

- 2 cups frozen wild blueberries
- 5 tablespoons chia seeds
- ¼ cup honey
- 1 tablespoon lemon or lime juice
- ¼ cup water
- 1½ cups all-purpose flour
- 1 cup whole-wheat flour
- ½ teaspoon salt
- 1 tablespoon sugar
- ½ cup cold unsalted butter
- 1 egg
- ½ cup plus 2 tablespoons milk, divided
- 1 cup powdered sugar
- 1 teaspoon vanilla extract

Directions:

1. To make the wild blueberry chia jam, place the blueberries, chia seeds, honey, lemon or lime juice, and water into a blender and pulse for 2 minutes. Pour the chia jam into a glass jar or bowl and cover. Store in the refrigerator at least 4 to 8 hours or until the jam is thickened.
2. In a food processor, place the all-purpose flour, whole-wheat flour, salt, sugar, and butter and process for 2 minutes, scraping down the sides of the food processor every 30 seconds. Add in the egg and blend for 30 seconds. Using the pulse button, add in ½ cup of the milk 1 tablespoon at a time or until the dough is moist enough to handle and be rolled into a ball. Let the dough rest at room temperature for 30 minutes.
3. On a floured surface, cut the dough in half; then form a ball and cut each ball into 6 equal pieces, totaling 12 equal pieces. Work with one piece at a time, and cover the remaining dough with a towel. Roll out the dough into a 6-inch round, much like a tortilla, with ¼ inch thickness. Place 4 tablespoons of filling in the center of round, fold over to form a half-circle. Using a fork, crimp the edges together and pierce the top with a fork for air holes. Repeat with the remaining dough and filling.
4. Preheat the air fryer to 350°F.
5. Working in batches, place 3 to 4 empanadas in the air fryer basket and spray with cooking spray. Cook for 8 minutes. Repeat in batches, as needed. Allow the sweet empanadas to cool for 15 minutes. Meanwhile, in a small bowl, whisk together the powdered sugar, the remaining 2 tablespoons of milk, and the vanilla extract. Then drizzle the glaze over the surface and serve.

Black And Blue Clafoutis

Servings: 2

Cooking Time: 15minutes

Ingredients:

- 6-inch pie pan
- 3 large eggs
- ½ cup sugar
- 1 teaspoon vanilla extract
- 2 tablespoons butter, melted 1 cup milk
- ½ cup all-purpose flour*
- 1 cup blackberries
- 1 cup blueberries
- 2 tablespoons confectioners' sugar

Directions:

1. Preheat the air fryer to 320°F.
2. Combine the eggs and sugar in a bowl and whisk vigorously until smooth, lighter in color and well combined. Add the vanilla extract, butter and milk and whisk together well. Add the flour and whisk just until no lumps or streaks of white remain.
3. Scatter half the blueberries and blackberries in a greased (6-inch) pie pan or cake pan. Pour half of the batter (about 1¼ cups) on top of the berries and transfer the tart pan to the air fryer basket. You can use an aluminum foil sling to help with this by taking a long piece of aluminum foil, folding it in half lengthwise twice until it is roughly 26-inches by 3-inches. Place this under the pie dish and hold the ends of the foil to move the pie dish in and out of the air fryer basket. Tuck the ends of the foil beside the pie dish while it cooks in the air fryer.
4. Air-fry at 320°F for 15 minutes or until the clafoutis has puffed up and is still a little jiggly in the center. Remove the clafoutis from the air fryer, invert it onto a plate and let it cool while you bake the second batch. Serve the clafoutis warm, dusted with confectioners' sugar on top.

Sweet Potato Pie Rolls

Servings:3

Cooking Time: 8 Minutes

Ingredients:

- 6 Spring roll wrappers
- 1½ cups Canned yams in syrup, drained
- 2 tablespoons Light brown sugar
- ¼ teaspoon Ground cinnamon
- 1 Large egg(s), well beaten
- Vegetable oil spray

Directions:

1. Preheat the air fryer to 400°F.
2. Set a spring roll wrapper on a clean, dry work surface. Scoop up ¼ cup of the pulpy yams and set along one edge of the wrapper, leaving 2 inches on each side of the yams. Top the yams with about 1 teaspoon brown sugar and a pinch of ground cinnamon. Fold the sides of the wrapper perpendicular to the yam filling up and over the filling, partially covering it. Brush beaten egg(s) over the side of the wrapper farthest from the yam. Starting with the yam end, roll the wrapper closed, ending at the part with the beaten egg that you can press gently to seal. Lightly coat the roll on all sides with vegetable oil spray. Set it aside seam side down and continue filling, rolling, and spraying the remaining wrappers in the same way.
3. Set the rolls seam side down in the basket with as much air space between them as possible. Air-fry undisturbed for 8 minutes, or until crisp and golden brown.
4. Use a nonstick-safe spatula and perhaps kitchen tongs for balance to gently transfer the rolls to a wire rack. Cool for at least 5 minutes or up to 30 minutes before serving.

One-bowl Chocolate Buttermilk Cake

Servings: 6

Cooking Time: 16-20 Minutes

Ingredients:

- ¾ cup All-purpose flour
- ½ cup Granulated white sugar
- 3 tablespoons Unsweetened cocoa powder
- ½ teaspoon Baking soda
- ¼ teaspoon Table salt
- ½ cup Buttermilk
- 2 tablespoons Vegetable oil
- ¾ teaspoon Vanilla extract
- Baking spray (see here)

Directions:

1. Preheat the air fryer to 325°F (or 330°F, if that's the closest setting).
2. Stir the flour, sugar, cocoa powder, baking soda, and salt in a large bowl until well combined. Add the buttermilk, oil, and vanilla. Stir just until a thick, grainy batter forms.
3. Use the baking spray to generously coat the inside of a 6-inch round cake pan for a small batch, a 7-inch round cake pan for a medium batch, or an 8-inch round cake pan for a large batch. Scrape and spread the chocolate batter into this pan, smoothing the batter out to an even layer.
4. Set the pan in the basket and air-fry undisturbed for 16 minutes for a 6-inch layer, 18 minutes for a 7-inch layer, or 20 minutes for an 8-inch layer, or until a toothpick or cake tester inserted into the center of the cake comes out clean. Start checking it at the 14-minute mark to know where you are.
5. Use hot pads or silicone baking mitts to transfer the cake pan to a wire rack. Cool for 5 minutes. To unmold, set a cutting board over the baking pan and invert both the board and the pan. Lift the still-warm pan off the cake layer. Set the wire rack on top of the cake layer and invert all of it with the cutting board so that the cake layer is now right side up on the wire rack. Remove the cutting board and continue cooling the cake for at least 10 minutes or to room temperature, about 30 minutes, before slicing into wedges.

Coconut Crusted Bananas With Pineapple Sauce

Servings: 4

Cooking Time: 5 Minutes

Ingredients:

- Pineapple Sauce
- 1½ cups puréed fresh pineapple
- 2 tablespoons sugar
- juice of 1 lemon
- ¼ teaspoon ground cinnamon
- 3 firm bananas
- ¼ cup sweetened condensed milk
- 1¼ cups shredded coconut
- ⅓ cup crushed graham crackers (crumbs)*
- vegetable or canola oil, in a spray bottle
- vanilla frozen yogurt or ice cream

Directions:

1. Make the pineapple sauce by combining the pineapple, sugar, lemon juice and cinnamon in a saucepan. Simmer the mixture on the stovetop for 20 minutes, and then set it aside.
2. Slice the bananas diagonally into ½-inch thick slices and place them in a bowl. Pour the sweetened condensed milk into the bowl and toss the bananas gently to coat. Combine the coconut and graham cracker crumbs together in a shallow dish. Remove the banana slices from the condensed milk and let any excess milk drip off. Dip the banana slices in the coconut and crumb mixture to coat both sides. Spray the coated slices with oil.
3. Preheat the air fryer to 400°F.
4. Grease the bottom of the air fryer basket with a little oil. Air-fry the bananas in batches at 400°F for 5 minutes, turning them over halfway through the cooking time. Air-fry until the bananas are golden brown on both sides.
5. Serve warm over vanilla frozen yogurt with some of the pineapple sauce spooned over top.

Boston Cream Donut Holes

Servings: 24

Cooking Time: 12 Minutes

Ingredients:

- 1½ cups bread flour
- 1 teaspoon active dry yeast
- 1 tablespoon sugar
- ¼ teaspoon salt
- ½ cup warm milk
- ½ teaspoon pure vanilla extract
- 2 egg yolks
- 2 tablespoons butter, melted
- vegetable oil
- Custard Filling:
- 1 (3.4-ounce) box French vanilla instant pudding mix
- ¾ cup whole milk
- ¼ cup heavy cream
- Chocolate Glaze:
- 1 cup chocolate chips
- ⅓ cup heavy cream

Directions:

1. Combine the flour, yeast, sugar and salt in the bowl of a stand mixer. Add the milk, vanilla, egg yolks and butter. Mix until the dough starts to come together in a ball. Transfer the dough to a floured surface and knead the dough by hand for 2 minutes. Shape the dough into a ball, place it in a large oiled bowl, cover the bowl with a clean kitchen towel and let the dough rise for 1 to 1½ hours or until the dough has doubled in size.
2. When the dough has risen, punch it down and roll it into a 24-inch log. Cut the dough into 24 pieces and roll each piece into a ball. Place the dough balls on a baking sheet and let them rise for another 30 minutes.
3. Preheat the air fryer to 400°F.
4. Spray or brush the dough balls lightly with vegetable oil and air-fry eight at a time for 4 minutes, turning them over halfway through the cooking time.
5. While donut holes are cooking, make the filling and chocolate glaze. To make the filling, use an electric hand mixer to beat the French vanilla pudding, milk and ¼ cup of heavy cream together for 2 minutes.
6. To make the chocolate glaze, place the chocolate chips in a medium-sized bowl. Bring the heavy cream to a boil on the stovetop and pour it over the chocolate chips. Stir until the chips are melted and the glaze is smooth.
7. To fill the donut holes, place the custard filling in a pastry bag with a long tip. Poke a hole into the side of the donut hole with a small knife. Wiggle the knife around to make room for the filling. Place the pastry bag tip into the hole and slowly squeeze the custard into the center of the donut. Dip the top half of the donut into the chocolate glaze, letting any excess glaze drip back into the bowl. Let the glazed donut holes sit for a few minutes before serving.

Chewy Coconut Cake

Servings: 6

Cooking Time: 18-22 Minutes

Ingredients:

- ¾ cup plus 2½ tablespoons All-purpose flour
- ¾ teaspoon Baking powder
- ⅛ teaspoon Table salt
- 7½ tablespoons (1 stick minus ½ tablespoon) Butter, at room temperature
- ⅓ cup plus 1 tablespoon Granulated white sugar
- 5 tablespoons Packed light brown sugar
- 5 tablespoons Pasteurized egg substitute, such as Egg Beaters
- 2 teaspoons Vanilla extract
- ½ cup Unsweetened shredded coconut (see here)
- Baking spray

Directions:

1. Preheat the air fryer to 325°F (or 330°F, if that's the closest setting).
2. Mix the flour, baking powder, and salt in a small bowl until well combined.
3. Using an electric hand mixer at medium speed , beat the butter, granulated white sugar, and brown sugar in a medium bowl until creamy and smooth, about 3 minutes, occasionally scraping down the inside of the bowl. Beat in the egg substitute or egg and vanilla until smooth.
4. Scrape down and remove the beaters. Fold in the flour mixture with a rubber spatula just until all the flour is moistened. Fold in the coconut until the mixture is a uniform color.
5. Use the baking spray to generously coat the inside of a 6-inch round cake pan for a small batch, a 7-inch round cake pan for a medium batch, or an 8-inch round cake pan for a large batch. Scrape and spread the batter into the pan, smoothing the batter out to an even layer.
6. Set the pan in the basket and air-fry for 18 minutes for a 6-inch layer, 20 minutes for a 7-inch layer, or 22 minutes for an 8-inch layer, or until the cake is well browned and set even if there's a little soft give right at the center. Start checking it at the 16-minute mark to know where you are.
7. Use hot pads or silicone baking mitts to transfer the cake pan to a wire rack. Cool for at least 1 hour or up to 4 hours. Use a nonstick-safe knife to slice the cake into wedges right in the pan, lifting them out one by one.

Sweet Potato Donut Holes

Servings: 18

Cooking Time: 4 Minutes Per Batch

Ingredients:

- 1 cup flour
- ⅓ cup sugar
- ¼ teaspoon baking soda
- 1 teaspoon baking powder
- ⅛ teaspoon salt
- ½ cup cooked mashed purple sweet potatoes
- 1 egg, beaten
- 2 tablespoons butter, melted
- 1 teaspoon pure vanilla extract
- oil for misting or cooking spray

Directions:

1. Preheat air fryer to 390°F.
2. In a large bowl, stir together the flour, sugar, baking soda, baking powder, and salt.
3. In a separate bowl, combine the potatoes, egg, butter, and vanilla and mix well.
4. Add potato mixture to dry ingredients and stir into a soft dough.
5. Shape dough into 1½-inch balls. Mist lightly with oil or cooking spray.
6. Place 9 donut holes in air fryer basket, leaving a little space in between. Cook for 4 minutes, until done in center and lightly browned outside.
7. Repeat step 6 to cook remaining donut holes.

Bread And Breakfast

Mediterranean Egg Sandwich

Servings: 1

Cooking Time: 8 Minutes

Ingredients:

- 1 large egg
- 5 baby spinach leaves, chopped
- 1 tablespoon roasted bell pepper, chopped
- 1 English muffin
- 1 thin slice prosciutto or Canadian bacon

Directions:

1. Spray a ramekin with cooking spray or brush the inside with extra-virgin olive oil.
2. In a small bowl, whisk together the egg, baby spinach, and bell pepper.
3. Split the English muffin in half and spray the inside lightly with cooking spray or brush with extra-virgin olive oil.
4. Preheat the air fryer to 350°F for 2 minutes. Place the egg ramekin and open English muffin into the air fryer basket, and cook at 350°F for 5 minutes. Open the air fryer drawer and add the prosciutto or bacon; cook for an additional 1 minute.
5. To assemble the sandwich, place the egg on one half of the English muffin, top with prosciutto or bacon, and place the remaining piece of English muffin on top.

Sweet-hot Pepperoni Pizza

Servings: 2

Cooking Time: 18 Minutes

Ingredients:

- 1 (6- to 8-ounce) pizza dough ball*
- olive oil
- ½ cup pizza sauce
- ¾ cup grated mozzarella cheese
- ½ cup thick sliced pepperoni
- ⅓ cup sliced pickled hot banana peppers
- ¼ teaspoon dried oregano
- 2 teaspoons honey

Directions:

1. Preheat the air fryer to 390°F.
2. Cut out a piece of aluminum foil the same size as the bottom of the air fryer basket. Brush the foil circle with olive oil. Shape the dough into a circle and place it on top of the foil. Dock the dough by piercing it several times with a fork. Brush the dough lightly with olive oil and transfer it into the air fryer basket with the foil on the bottom.
3. Air-fry the plain pizza dough for 6 minutes. Turn the dough over, remove the aluminum foil and brush again with olive oil. Air-fry for an additional 4 minutes.
4. Spread the pizza sauce on top of the dough and sprinkle the mozzarella cheese over the sauce. Top with the pepperoni, pepper slices and dried oregano. Lower the temperature of the air fryer to 350°F and cook for 8 minutes, until the cheese has melted and lightly browned. Transfer the pizza to a cutting board and drizzle with the honey. Slice and serve.

Peppered Maple Bacon Knots

Servings: 6

Cooking Time: 8 Minutes

Ingredients:

- 1 pound maple smoked center-cut bacon
- ¼ cup maple syrup
- ¼ cup brown sugar
- coarsely cracked black peppercorns

Directions:

1. Tie each bacon strip in a loose knot and place them on a baking sheet.
2. Combine the maple syrup and brown sugar in a bowl. Brush each knot generously with this mixture and sprinkle with coarsely cracked black pepper.
3. Preheat the air fryer to 390°F.
4. Air-fry the bacon knots in batches. Place one layer of knots in the air fryer basket and air-fry for 5 minutes. Turn the bacon knots over and air-fry for an additional 3 minutes.
5. Serve warm.

Chocolate Chip Banana Muffins

Servings: 12

Cooking Time: 14 Minutes

Ingredients:

- 2 medium bananas, mashed
- ¼ cup brown sugar
- 1½ teaspoons vanilla extract
- ⅔ cup milk
- 2 tablespoons butter
- 1 large egg
- 1 cup white whole-wheat flour
- ½ cup old-fashioned oats
- 1 teaspoon baking soda
- ½ teaspoon baking powder
- ⅛ teaspoon sea salt
- ¼ cup mini chocolate chips

Directions:

1. Preheat the air fryer to 330°F.
2. In a large bowl, combine the bananas, brown sugar, vanilla extract, milk, butter, and egg; set aside.
3. In a separate bowl, combine the flour, oats, baking soda, baking powder, and salt.
4. Slowly add the dry ingredients into the wet ingredients, folding in the flour mixture ⅓ cup at a time.
5. Mix in the chocolate chips and set aside.
6. Using silicone muffin liners, fill 6 muffin liners two-thirds full. Carefully place the muffin liners in the air fryer basket and bake for 20 minutes (or until the tops are browned and a toothpick inserted in the center comes out clean). Carefully remove the muffins from the basket and repeat with the remaining batter.
7. Serve warm.

Apple Fritters

Servings: 6

Cooking Time: 12 Minutes

Ingredients:

- 1 cup all-purpose flour
- 1½ teaspoons baking powder
- ¼ teaspoon salt
- 2 tablespoon brown sugar
- 1 teaspoon vanilla extract
- ¾ cup plain Greek yogurt
- 1 tablespoon cinnamon
- 1 large Granny Smith apple, cored, peeled, and finely chopped
- ¼ cup chopped walnuts
- ½ cup powdered sugar
- 1 tablespoon milk

Directions:

1. Preheat the air fryer to 320°F.
2. In a medium bowl, combine the flour, baking powder, and salt.
3. In a large bowl, add the brown sugar, vanilla, yogurt, cinnamon, apples, and walnuts. Mix the dry ingredients into the wet, using your hands to combine, until all the ingredients are mixed together. Knead the mixture in the bowl about 4 times.
4. Lightly spray the air fryer basket with olive oil spray.
5. Divide the batter into 6 equally sized balls; then lightly flatten them and place inside the basket. Repeat until all the fritters are formed.
6. Place the basket in the air fryer and cook for 6 minutes, flip, and then cook another 6 minutes.
7. While the fritters are cooking, in a small bowl, mix the powdered sugar with the milk. Set aside.
8. When the cooking completes, remove the air fryer basket and allow the fritters to cool on a wire rack. Drizzle with the homemade glaze and serve.

French Toast Sticks

Servings: 4

Cooking Time: 7 Minutes

Ingredients:

- 2 eggs
- ½ cup milk
- ⅛ teaspoon salt
- ½ teaspoon pure vanilla extract
- ¾ cup crushed cornflakes
- 6 slices sandwich bread, each slice cut into 4 strips
- oil for misting or cooking spray
- maple syrup or honey

Directions:

1. In a small bowl, beat together eggs, milk, salt, and vanilla.
2. Place crushed cornflakes on a plate or in a shallow dish.
3. Dip bread strips in egg mixture, shake off excess, and roll in cornflake crumbs.
4. Spray both sides of bread strips with oil.
5. Place bread strips in air fryer basket in single layer.
6. Cook at 390°F for 7minutes or until they're dark golden brown.
7. Repeat steps 5 and 6 to cook remaining French toast sticks.
8. Serve with maple syrup or honey for dipping.

Crispy Bacon

Servings: 6

Cooking Time: 20 Minutes

Ingredients:

- 12 ounces bacon

Directions:

1. Preheat the air fryer to 350°F for 3 minutes.
2. Lay out the bacon in a single layer, slightly overlapping the strips of bacon.
3. Air fry for 10 minutes or until desired crispness.
4. Repeat until all the bacon has been cooked.

Whole-grain Cornbread

Servings: 6

Cooking Time: 25 Minutes

Ingredients:

- 1 cup stoneground cornmeal
- ½ cup brown rice flour
- 1 teaspoon sugar
- 2 teaspoons baking powder
- ¼ teaspoon salt
- 1 cup milk
- 2 tablespoons oil
- 2 eggs
- cooking spray

Directions:

1. Preheat the air fryer to 360°F.
2. In a medium mixing bowl, mix cornmeal, brown rice flour, sugar, baking powder, and salt together.
3. Add the remaining ingredients and beat with a spoon until batter is smooth.
4. Spray air fryer baking pan with nonstick cooking spray and add the cornbread batter.
5. Bake at 360°F for 25 minutes, until center is done.

Crustless Broccoli, Roasted Pepper And Fontina Quiche

Servings: 4

Cooking Time: 60 Minutes

Ingredients:

- 7-inch cake pan
- 1 cup broccoli florets
- ¾ cup chopped roasted red peppers
- 1¼ cups grated Fontina cheese
- 6 eggs
- ¾ cup heavy cream
- ½ teaspoon salt
- freshly ground black pepper

Directions:

1. Preheat the air fryer to 360°F.
2. Grease the inside of a 7-inch cake pan (4 inches deep) or other oven-safe pan that will fit into your air fryer. Place the broccoli florets and roasted red peppers in the cake pan and top with the grated Fontina cheese.
3. Whisk the eggs and heavy cream together in a bowl. Season the eggs with salt and freshly ground black pepper. Pour the egg mixture over the cheese and vegetables and cover the pan with aluminum foil. Transfer the cake pan to the air fryer basket.
4. Air-fry at 360°F for 60 minutes. Remove the aluminum foil for the last two minutes of cooking time.
5. Unmold the quiche onto a platter and cut it into slices to serve with a side salad or perhaps some air-fried potatoes.

Zucchini Walnut Bread

Servings: 6

Cooking Time: 30 Minutes

Ingredients:

- ¾ cup all-purpose flour
- ½ teaspoon baking soda
- 1 teaspoon ground cinnamon
- ⅛ teaspoon salt
- 1 large egg
- ⅓ cup packed brown sugar
- ¼ cup canola oil
- 1 teaspoon vanilla extract
- ⅓ cup milk
- 1 medium zucchini, shredded (about 1⅓ cups)
- ⅓ cup chopped walnuts

Directions:

1. Preheat the air fryer to 320°F.
2. In a medium bowl, mix together the flour, baking soda, cinnamon, and salt.
3. In a large bowl, whisk together the egg, brown sugar, oil, vanilla, and milk. Stir in the zucchini.
4. Slowly fold the dry ingredients into the wet ingredients. Stir in the chopped walnuts. Then pour the batter into two 4-inch oven-safe loaf pans.
5. Bake for 30 minutes or until a toothpick inserted into the center comes out clean. Let cool before slicing.
6. NOTE: Store tightly wrapped on the counter for up to 5 days, in the refrigerator for up to 10 days, or in the freezer for 3 months.

Vegetarians Recipes

Pinto Taquitos

Servings: 4

Cooking Time: 8 Minutes

Ingredients:

- 12 corn tortillas (6- to 7-inch size)
- Filling
- ½ cup refried pinto beans
- ½ cup grated sharp Cheddar or Pepper Jack cheese
- ¼ cup corn kernels (if frozen, measure after thawing and draining)
- 2 tablespoons chopped green onion
- 2 tablespoons chopped jalapeño pepper (seeds and ribs removed before chopping)
- ½ teaspoon lime juice
- ½ teaspoon chile powder, plus extra for dusting
- ½ teaspoon cumin
- ½ teaspoon garlic powder
- oil for misting or cooking spray
- salsa, sour cream, or guacamole for dipping

Directions:

1. Mix together all filling Ingredients.
2. Warm refrigerated tortillas for easier rolling. (Wrap in damp paper towels and microwave for 30 to 60 seconds.)
3. Working with one at a time, place 1 tablespoon of filling on tortilla and roll up. Spray with oil or cooking spray and dust outside with chile powder to taste.
4. Place 6 taquitos in air fryer basket (4 on bottom layer, 2 stacked crosswise on top). Cook at 390°F for 8 minutes, until crispy and brown.
5. Repeat step 4 to cook remaining taquitos.
6. Serve plain or with salsa, sour cream, or guacamole for dipping.

Charred Cauliflower Tacos

Servings: 4

Cooking Time: 10 Minutes

Ingredients:

- 1 head cauliflower, washed and cut into florets
- 2 tablespoons avocado oil
- 2 teaspoons taco seasoning
- 1 medium avocado
- ½ teaspoon garlic powder
- ¼ teaspoon black pepper
- ¼ teaspoon salt
- 2 tablespoons chopped red onion
- 2 teaspoons fresh squeezed lime juice
- ¼ cup chopped cilantro
- Eight 6-inch corn tortillas
- ½ cup cooked corn
- ½ cup shredded purple cabbage

Directions:

1. Preheat the air fryer to 390°F.
2. In a large bowl, toss the cauliflower with the avocado oil and taco seasoning. Set the metal trivet inside the air fryer basket and liberally spray with olive oil.
3. Place the cauliflower onto the trivet and cook for 10 minutes, shaking every 3 minutes to allow for an even char.
4. While the cauliflower is cooking, prepare the avocado sauce. In a medium bowl, mash the avocado; then mix in the garlic powder, pepper, salt, and onion. Stir in the lime juice and cilantro; set aside.
5. Remove the cauliflower from the air fryer basket.
6. Place 1 tablespoon of avocado sauce in the middle of a tortilla, and top with corn, cabbage, and charred cauliflower. Repeat with the remaining tortillas. Serve immediately.

Spicy Sesame Tempeh Slaw With Peanut Dressing

Servings: 2

Cooking Time: 8 Minutes

Ingredients:

- 2 cups hot water
- 1 teaspoon salt
- 8 ounces tempeh, sliced into 1-inch-long pieces
- 2 tablespoons low-sodium soy sauce
- 2 tablespoons rice vinegar
- 1 tablespoon filtered water
- 2 teaspoons sesame oil
- ½ teaspoon fresh ginger
- 1 clove garlic, minced
- ¼ teaspoon black pepper
- ½ jalapeño, sliced
- 4 cups cabbage slaw
- 4 tablespoons Peanut Dressing (see the following recipe)
- 2 tablespoons fresh chopped cilantro
- 2 tablespoons chopped peanuts

Directions:

1. Mix the hot water with the salt and pour over the tempeh in a glass bowl. Stir and cover with a towel for 10 minutes.
2. Discard the water and leave the tempeh in the bowl.
3. In a medium bowl, mix the soy sauce, rice vinegar, filtered water, sesame oil, ginger, garlic, pepper, and jalapeño. Pour over the tempeh and cover with a towel. Place in the refrigerator to marinate for at least 2 hours.
4. Preheat the air fryer to 370°F. Remove the tempeh from the bowl and discard the remaining marinade.
5. Liberally spray the metal trivet that goes into the air fryer basket and place the tempeh on top of the trivet.
6. Cook for 4 minutes, flip, and cook another 4 minutes.
7. In a large bowl, mix the cabbage slaw with the Peanut Dressing and toss in the cilantro and chopped peanuts.
8. Portion onto 4 plates and place the cooked tempeh on top when cooking completes. Serve immediately.

Spaghetti Squash And Kale Fritters With Pomodoro Sauce

Servings: 3

Cooking Time: 45 Minutes

Ingredients:

- 1½-pound spaghetti squash (about half a large or a whole small squash)
- olive oil
- ½ onion, diced
- ½ red bell pepper, diced
- 2 cloves garlic, minced
- 4 cups coarsely chopped kale
- salt and freshly ground black pepper
- 1 egg
- ⅓ cup breadcrumbs, divided*
- ⅓ cup grated Parmesan cheese
- ½ teaspoon dried rubbed sage
- pinch nutmeg
- Pomodoro Sauce:
- 2 tablespoons olive oil
- ½ onion, chopped
- 1 to 2 cloves garlic, minced
- 1 (28-ounce) can peeled tomatoes
- ¼ cup red wine
- 1 teaspoon Italian seasoning
- 2 tablespoons chopped fresh basil, plus more for garnish
- salt and freshly ground black pepper
- ½ teaspoon sugar (optional)

Directions:

1. Preheat the air fryer to 370°F.
2. Cut the spaghetti squash in half lengthwise and remove the seeds. Rub the inside of the squash with olive oil and season with salt and pepper. Place the squash, cut side up, into the air fryer basket and air-fry for 30 minutes, flipping the squash over halfway through the cooking process.
3. While the squash is cooking, Preheat a large sauté pan over medium heat on the stovetop. Add a little olive oil and sauté the onions for 3 minutes, until they start to soften. Add the red pepper and garlic and continue to sauté for an additional 4 minutes. Add the kale and season with salt and pepper. Cook for 2 more minutes, or until the kale is soft. Transfer the mixture to a large bowl and let it cool.
4. While the squash continues to cook, make the Pomodoro sauce. Preheat the large sauté pan again over medium heat on the stovetop. Add the olive oil and sauté the onion and garlic for 2 to 3 minutes, until the onion begins to soften. Crush the canned tomatoes with your hands and add them to the pan along with the red wine and Italian seasoning and simmer for 20 minutes. Add the basil and season to taste with salt, pepper and sugar (if using).
5. When the spaghetti squash has finished cooking, use a fork to scrape the inside flesh of the squash onto a sheet pan. Spread the squash out and let it cool.
6. Once cool, add the spaghetti squash to the kale mixture, along with the egg, breadcrumbs, Parmesan cheese, sage, nutmeg, salt and freshly ground black pepper. Stir to combine well and then divide the

mixture into 6 thick portions. You can shape the portions into patties, but I prefer to keep them a little random and unique in shape. Spray or brush the fritters with olive oil.

7. Preheat the air fryer to 370°F.
8. Brush the air fryer basket with a little olive oil and transfer the fritters to the basket. Air-fry the squash and kale fritters at 370°F for 15 minutes, flipping them over halfway through the cooking process.
9. Serve the fritters warm with the Pomodoro sauce spooned over the top or pooled on your plate. Garnish with the fresh basil leaves.

Basic Fried Tofu

Servings: 4

Cooking Time: 17 Minutes

Ingredients:

- 14 ounces extra-firm tofu, drained and pressed
- 1 tablespoon sesame oil
- 2 tablespoons low-sodium soy sauce
- ¼ cup rice vinegar
- 1 tablespoon fresh grated ginger
- 1 clove garlic, minced
- 3 tablespoons cornstarch
- ¼ teaspoon black pepper
- ⅛ teaspoon salt

Directions:

1. Cut the tofu into 16 cubes. Set aside in a glass container with a lid.
2. In a medium bowl, mix the sesame oil, soy sauce, rice vinegar, ginger, and garlic. Pour over the tofu and secure the lid. Place in the refrigerator to marinate for an hour.
3. Preheat the air fryer to 350°F.
4. In a small bowl, mix the cornstarch, black pepper, and salt.
5. Transfer the tofu to a large bowl and discard the leftover marinade. Pour the cornstarch mixture over the tofu and toss until all the pieces are coated.
6. Liberally spray the air fryer basket with olive oil mist and set the tofu pieces inside. Allow space between the tofu so it can cook evenly. Cook in batches if necessary.
7. Cook 15 to 17 minutes, shaking the basket every 5 minutes to allow the tofu to cook evenly on all sides. When it's done cooking, the tofu will be crisped and browned on all sides.
8. Remove the tofu from the air fryer basket and serve warm.

Pizza Portobello Mushrooms

Servings: 2

Cooking Time: 18 Minutes

Ingredients:

- 2 portobello mushroom caps, gills removed (see Figure 13-1)
- 1 teaspoon extra-virgin olive oil
- ¼ cup diced onion
- 1 teaspoon minced garlic
- 1 medium zucchini, shredded
- 1 teaspoon dried oregano
- ½ teaspoon black pepper
- ¼ teaspoon salt
- ⅓ cup marinara sauce
- ¼ cup shredded part-skim mozzarella cheese
- ¼ teaspoon red pepper flakes
- 2 tablespoons Parmesan cheese
- 2 tablespoons chopped basil

Directions:

1. Preheat the air fryer to 370°F.
2. Lightly spray the mushrooms with an olive oil mist and place into the air fryer to cook for 10 minutes, cap side up.
3. Add the olive oil to a pan and sauté the onion and garlic together for about 2 to 4 minutes. Stir in the zucchini, oregano, pepper, and salt, and continue to cook. When the zucchini has cooked down (usually about 4 to 6 minutes), add in the marinara sauce. Remove from the heat and stir in the mozzarella cheese.
4. Remove the mushrooms from the air fryer basket when cooking completes. Reset the temperature to 350°F.
5. Using a spoon, carefully stuff the mushrooms with the zucchini marinara mixture.
6. Return the stuffed mushrooms to the air fryer basket and cook for 5 to 8 minutes, or until the cheese is lightly browned. You should be able to easily insert a fork into the mushrooms when they're cooked.
7. Remove the mushrooms and sprinkle the red pepper flakes, Parmesan cheese, and fresh basil over the top.
8. Serve warm.

Stuffed Zucchini Boats

Servings: 2

Cooking Time: 20 Minutes

Ingredients:

- olive oil
- ½ cup onion, finely chopped
- 1 clove garlic, finely minced
- ½ teaspoon dried oregano
- ¼ teaspoon dried thyme
- ¾ cup couscous
- 1½ cups chicken stock, divided
- 1 tomato, seeds removed and finely chopped
- ½ cup coarsely chopped Kalamata olives
- ½ cup grated Romano cheese
- ¼ cup pine nuts, toasted
- 1 tablespoon chopped fresh parsley
- 1 teaspoon salt
- freshly ground black pepper
- 1 egg, beaten
- 1 cup grated mozzarella cheese, divided
- 2 thick zucchini

Directions:

1. Preheat a sauté pan on the stovetop over medium-high heat. Add the olive oil and sauté the onion until it just starts to soften–about 4 minutes. Stir in the garlic, dried oregano and thyme. Add the couscous and sauté for just a minute. Add 1¼ cups of the chicken stock and simmer over low heat for 3 to 5 minutes, until liquid has been absorbed and the couscous is soft. Remove the pan from heat and set it aside to cool slightly.
2. Fluff the couscous and add the tomato, Kalamata olives, Romano cheese, pine nuts, parsley, salt and pepper. Mix well. Add the remaining chicken stock, the egg and ½ cup of the mozzarella cheese. Stir to ensure everything is combined.
3. Cut each zucchini in half lengthwise. Then, trim each half of the zucchini into four 5-inch lengths. (Save the trimmed ends of the zucchini for another use.) Use a spoon to scoop out the center of the zucchini, leaving some flesh around the sides. Brush both sides of the zucchini with olive oil and season the cut side with salt and pepper.
4. Preheat the air fryer to 380°F.
5. Divide the couscous filling between the four zucchini boats. Use your hands to press the filling together and fill the inside of the zucchini. The filling should be mounded into the boats and rounded on top.
6. Transfer the zucchini boats to the air fryer basket and drizzle the stuffed zucchini boats with olive oil. Air-fry for 19 minutes. Then, sprinkle the remaining mozzarella cheese on top of the zucchini, pressing it down onto the filling lightly to prevent it from blowing around in the air fryer. Air-fry for one more minute to melt the cheese. Transfer the finished zucchini boats to a serving platter and garnish with the chopped parsley.

Roasted Vegetable Pita Pizza

Servings: 4

Cooking Time: 20 Minutes

Ingredients:

- 1 medium red bell pepper, seeded and cut into quarters
- 1 teaspoon extra-virgin olive oil
- ⅛ teaspoon black pepper
- ⅛ teaspoon salt
- Two 6-inch whole-grain pita breads
- 6 tablespoons pesto sauce
- ¼ small red onion, thinly sliced
- ½ cup shredded part-skim mozzarella cheese

Directions:

1. Preheat the air fryer to 400°F.
2. In a small bowl, toss the bell peppers with the olive oil, pepper, and salt.
3. Place the bell peppers in the air fryer and cook for 15 minutes, shaking every 5 minutes to prevent burning.
4. Remove the peppers and set aside. Turn the air fryer temperature down to 350°F.
5. Lay the pita bread on a flat surface. Cover each with half the pesto sauce; then top with even portions of the red bell peppers and onions. Sprinkle cheese over the top. Spray the air fryer basket with olive oil mist.
6. Carefully lift the pita bread into the air fryer basket with a spatula.
7. Cook for 5 to 8 minutes, or until the outer edges begin to brown and the cheese is melted.
8. Serve warm with desired sides.

Rigatoni With Roasted Onions, Fennel, Spinach And Lemon Pepper Ricotta

Servings: 2

Cooking Time: 13 Minutes

Ingredients:

- 1 red onion, rough chopped into large chunks
- 2 teaspoons olive oil, divided
- 1 bulb fennel, sliced ¼-inch thick
- ¾ cup ricotta cheese
- 1½ teaspoons finely chopped lemon zest, plus more for garnish
- 1 teaspoon lemon juice
- salt and freshly ground black pepper
- 8 ounces (½ pound) dried rigatoni pasta
- 3 cups baby spinach leaves

Directions:

1. Bring a large stockpot of salted water to a boil on the stovetop and Preheat the air fryer to 400°F.
2. While the water is coming to a boil, toss the chopped onion in 1 teaspoon of olive oil and transfer to the air fryer basket. Air-fry at 400°F for 5 minutes. Toss the sliced fennel with 1 teaspoon of olive oil and add this to the air fryer basket with the onions. Continue to air-fry at 400°F for 8 minutes, shaking the basket a few times during the cooking process.
3. Combine the ricotta cheese, lemon zest and juice, ¼ teaspoon of salt and freshly ground black pepper in a bowl and stir until smooth.
4. Add the dried rigatoni to the boiling water and cook according to the package directions. When the pasta is cooked al dente, reserve one cup of the pasta water and drain the pasta into a colander.
5. Place the spinach in a serving bowl and immediately transfer the hot pasta to the bowl, wilting the spinach. Add the roasted onions and fennel and toss together. Add a little pasta water to the dish if it needs moistening. Then, dollop the lemon pepper ricotta cheese on top and nestle it into the hot pasta. Garnish with more lemon zest if desired.

Falafel

Servings: 4

Cooking Time: 10 Minutes

Ingredients:

- 1 cup dried chickpeas
- ½ onion, chopped
- 1 clove garlic
- ¼ cup fresh parsley leaves
- 1 teaspoon salt
- ¼ teaspoon crushed red pepper flakes
- 1 teaspoon ground cumin
- ½ teaspoon ground coriander
- 1 to 2 tablespoons flour
- olive oil
- Tomato Salad
- 2 tomatoes, seeds removed and diced
- ½ cucumber, finely diced
- ¼ red onion, finely diced and rinsed with water
- 1 teaspoon red wine vinegar
- 1 tablespoon olive oil
- salt and freshly ground black pepper
- 2 tablespoons chopped fresh parsley

Directions:

1. Cover the chickpeas with water and let them soak overnight on the counter. Then drain the chickpeas and put them in a food processor, along with the onion, garlic, parsley, spices and 1 tablespoon of flour. Pulse in the food processor until the mixture has broken down into a coarse paste consistency. The mixture should hold together when you pinch it. Add more flour as needed, until you get this consistency.
2. Scoop portions of the mixture (about 2 tablespoons in size) and shape into balls. Place the balls on a plate and refrigerate for at least 30 minutes. You should have between 12 and 14 balls.
3. Preheat the air fryer to 380°F.
4. Spray the falafel balls with oil and place them in the air fryer. Air-fry for 10 minutes, rolling them over and spraying them with oil again halfway through the cooking time so that they cook and brown evenly.
5. Serve with pita bread, hummus, cucumbers, hot peppers, tomatoes or any other fillings you might like.

Sandwiches And Burgers Recipes

Lamb Burgers

Servings: 3

Cooking Time: 17 Minutes

Ingredients:

- 1 pound 2 ounces Ground lamb
- 3 tablespoons Crumbled feta
- 1 teaspoon Minced garlic
- 1 teaspoon Tomato paste
- ¾ teaspoon Ground coriander
- ¾ teaspoon Ground dried ginger
- Up to ⅛ teaspoon Cayenne
- Up to a ⅛ teaspoon Table salt (optional)
- 3 Kaiser rolls or hamburger buns (gluten-free, if a concern), split open

Directions:

1. Preheat the air fryer to 375°F .
2. Gently mix the ground lamb, feta, garlic, tomato paste, coriander, ginger, cayenne, and salt (if using) in a bowl until well combined, trying to keep the bits of cheese intact. Form this mixture into two 5-inch patties for the small batch, three 5-inch patties for the medium, or four 5-inch patties for the large.
3. Set the patties in the basket in one layer and air-fry undisturbed for 16 minutes, or until an instant-read meat thermometer inserted into one burger registers 160°F. (The cheese is not an issue with the temperature probe in this recipe as it was for the Inside-Out Cheeseburgers, because the feta is so well mixed into the ground meat.)
4. Use a nonstick-safe spatula, and perhaps a flatware fork for balance, to transfer the burgers to a cutting board. Set the buns cut side down in the basket in one layer (working in batches as necessary) and air-fry undisturbed for 1 minute, to toast a bit and warm up. Serve the burgers warm in the buns.

Chicken Spiedies

Servings: 3

Cooking Time: 12 Minutes

Ingredients:

- 1¼ pounds Boneless skinless chicken thighs, trimmed of any fat blobs and cut into 2-inch pieces
- 3 tablespoons Red wine vinegar
- 2 tablespoons Olive oil
- 2 tablespoons Minced fresh mint leaves
- 2 tablespoons Minced fresh parsley leaves
- 2 teaspoons Minced fresh dill fronds
- ¾ teaspoon Fennel seeds
- ¾ teaspoon Table salt
- Up to a ¼ teaspoon Red pepper flakes
- 3 Long soft rolls, such as hero, hoagie, or Italian sub rolls (gluten-free, if a concern), split open lengthwise
- 4½ tablespoons Regular or low-fat mayonnaise (not fat-free; gluten-free, if a concern)
- 1½ tablespoons Distilled white vinegar
- 1½ teaspoons Ground black pepper

Directions:

1. Mix the chicken, vinegar, oil, mint, parsley, dill, fennel seeds, salt, and red pepper flakes in a zip-closed plastic bag. Seal, gently massage the marinade ingredients into the meat, and refrigerate for at least 2 hours or up to 6 hours. (Longer than that and the meat can turn rubbery.)
2. Set the plastic bag out on the counter (to make the contents a little less frigid). Preheat the air fryer to 400°F.
3. When the machine is at temperature, use kitchen tongs to set the chicken thighs in the basket (discard any remaining marinade) and air-fry undisturbed for 6 minutes. Turn the thighs over and continue air-frying undisturbed for 6 minutes more, until well browned, cooked through, and even a little crunchy.
4. Dump the contents of the basket onto a wire rack and cool for 2 or 3 minutes. Divide the chicken evenly between the rolls. Whisk the mayonnaise, vinegar, and black pepper in a small bowl until smooth. Drizzle this sauce over the chicken pieces in the rolls.

Thanksgiving Turkey Sandwiches

Servings: 3

Cooking Time: 10 Minutes

Ingredients:

- 1½ cups Herb-seasoned stuffing mix (not cornbread-style; gluten-free, if a concern)
- 1 Large egg white(s)
- 2 tablespoons Water
- 3 5- to 6-ounce turkey breast cutlets
- Vegetable oil spray
- 4½ tablespoons Purchased cranberry sauce, preferably whole berry
- ⅛ teaspoon Ground cinnamon
- ⅛ teaspoon Ground dried ginger
- 4½ tablespoons Regular, low-fat, or fat-free mayonnaise (gluten-free, if a concern)
- 6 tablespoons Shredded Brussels sprouts
- 3 Kaiser rolls (gluten-free, if a concern), split open

Directions:

1. Preheat the air fryer to 375°F .
2. Put the stuffing mix in a heavy zip-closed bag, seal it, lay it flat on your counter, and roll a rolling pin over the bag to crush the stuffing mix to the consistency of rough sand. (Or you can pulse the stuffing mix to the desired consistency in a food processor.)
3. Set up and fill two shallow soup plates or small pie plates on your counter: one for the egg white(s), whisked with the water until foamy; and one for the ground stuffing mix.
4. Dip a cutlet in the egg white mixture, coating both sides and letting any excess egg white slip back into the rest. Set the cutlet in the ground stuffing mix and coat it evenly on both sides, pressing gently to coat well on both sides. Lightly coat the cutlet on both sides with vegetable oil spray, set it aside, and continue dipping and coating the remaining cutlets in the same way.
5. Set the cutlets in the basket and air-fry undisturbed for 10 minutes, or until crisp and brown. Use kitchen tongs to transfer the cutlets to a wire rack to cool for a few minutes.
6. Meanwhile, stir the cranberry sauce with the cinnamon and ginger in a small bowl. Mix the shredded Brussels sprouts and mayonnaise in a second bowl until the vegetable is evenly coated.
7. Build the sandwiches by spreading about 1½ tablespoons of the cranberry mixture on the cut side of the bottom half of each roll. Set a cutlet on top, then spread about 3 tablespoons of the Brussels sprouts mixture evenly over the cutlet. Set the other half of the roll on top and serve warm.

Chicken Gyros

Servings: 4

Cooking Time: 14 Minutes

Ingredients:

- 4 4- to 5-ounce boneless skinless chicken thighs, trimmed of any fat blobs
- 2 tablespoons Lemon juice
- 2 tablespoons Red wine vinegar
- 2 tablespoons Olive oil
- 2 teaspoons Dried oregano
- 2 teaspoons Minced garlic
- 1 teaspoon Table salt
- 1 teaspoon Ground black pepper
- 4 Pita pockets (gluten-free, if a concern)
- ½ cup Chopped tomatoes
- ½ cup Bottled regular, low-fat, or fat-free ranch dressing (gluten-free, if a concern)

Directions:

1. Mix the thighs, lemon juice, vinegar, oil, oregano, garlic, salt, and pepper in a zip-closed bag. Seal, gently massage the marinade into the meat through the plastic, and refrigerate for at least 2 hours or up to 6 hours. (Longer than that and the meat can turn rubbery.)
2. Set the plastic bag out on the counter (to make the contents a little less frigid). Preheat the air fryer to 375°F .
3. When the machine is at temperature, use kitchen tongs to place the thighs in the basket in one layer. Discard the marinade. Air-fry the chicken thighs undisturbed for 12 minutes, or until browned and an instant-read meat thermometer inserted into the thickest part of one thigh registers 165°F. You may need to air-fry the chicken 2 minutes longer if the machine's temperature is 360°F.
4. Use kitchen tongs to transfer the thighs to a cutting board. Cool for 5 minutes, then set one thigh in each of the pita pockets. Top each with 2 tablespoons chopped tomatoes and 2 tablespoons dressing. Serve warm.

Best-ever Roast Beef Sandwiches

Servings: 6

Cooking Time: 30-50 Minutes

Ingredients:

- 2½ teaspoons Olive oil
- 1½ teaspoons Dried oregano
- 1½ teaspoons Dried thyme
- 1½ teaspoons Onion powder
- 1½ teaspoons Table salt
- 1½ teaspoons Ground black pepper
- 3 pounds Beef eye of round
- 6 Round soft rolls, such as Kaiser rolls or hamburger buns (gluten-free, if a concern), split open lengthwise
- ¾ cup Regular, low-fat, or fat-free mayonnaise (gluten-free, if a concern)
- 6 Romaine lettuce leaves, rinsed
- 6 Round tomato slices (¼ inch thick)

Directions:

1. Preheat the air fryer to 350°F .
2. Mix the oil, oregano, thyme, onion powder, salt, and pepper in a small bowl. Spread this mixture all over the eye of round.
3. When the machine is at temperature, set the beef in the basket and air-fry for 30 to 50 minutes (the range depends on the size of the cut), turning the meat twice, until an instant-read meat thermometer inserted into the thickest piece of the meat registers 130°F for rare, 140°F for medium, or 150°F for well-done.
4. Use kitchen tongs to transfer the beef to a cutting board. Cool for 10 minutes. If serving now, carve into ⅛-inch-thick slices. Spread each roll with 2 tablespoons mayonnaise and divide the beef slices between the rolls. Top with a lettuce leaf and a tomato slice and serve. Or set the beef in a container, cover, and refrigerate for up to 3 days to make cold roast beef sandwiches anytime.

Crunchy Falafel Balls

Servings: 8

Cooking Time: 16 Minutes

Ingredients:

- 2½ cups Drained and rinsed canned chickpeas
- ¼ cup Olive oil
- 3 tablespoons All-purpose flour
- 1½ teaspoons Dried oregano
- 1½ teaspoons Dried sage leaves
- 1½ teaspoons Dried thyme
- ¾ teaspoon Table salt
- Olive oil spray

Directions:

1. Preheat the air fryer to 400°F.
2. Place the chickpeas, olive oil, flour, oregano, sage, thyme, and salt in a food processor. Cover and process into a paste, stopping the machine at least once to scrape down the inside of the canister.
3. Scrape down and remove the blade. Using clean, wet hands, form 2 tablespoons of the paste into a ball, then continue making 9 more balls for a small batch, 15 more for a medium one, and 19 more for a large batch. Generously coat the balls in olive oil spray.
4. Set the balls in the basket in one layer with a little space between them and air-fry undisturbed for 16 minutes, or until well browned and crisp.
5. Dump the contents of the basket onto a wire rack. Cool for 5 minutes before serving.

Sausage And Pepper Heros

Servings: 3

Cooking Time: 11 Minutes

Ingredients:

- 3 links (about 9 ounces total) Sweet Italian sausages (gluten-free, if a concern)
- 1½ Medium red or green bell pepper(s), stemmed, cored, and cut into ½-inch-wide strips
- 1 medium Yellow or white onion(s), peeled, halved, and sliced into thin half-moons
- 3 Long soft rolls, such as hero, hoagie, or Italian sub rolls (gluten-free, if a concern), split open lengthwise
- For garnishing Balsamic vinegar
- For garnishing Fresh basil leaves

Directions:

1. Preheat the air fryer to 400°F.
2. When the machine is at temperature, set the sausage links in the basket in one layer and air-fry undisturbed for 5 minutes.
3. Add the pepper strips and onions. Continue air-frying, tossing and rearranging everything about once every minute, for 5 minutes, or until the sausages are browned and an instant-read meat thermometer inserted into one of the links registers 160°F.
4. Use a nonstick-safe spatula and kitchen tongs to transfer the sausages and vegetables to a cutting board. Set the rolls cut side down in the basket in one layer (working in batches as necessary) and air-fry undisturbed for 1 minute, to toast the rolls a bit and warm them up. Set 1 sausage with some pepper strips and onions in each warm roll, sprinkle balsamic vinegar over the sandwich fillings, and garnish with basil leaves.

Black Bean Veggie Burgers

Servings: 3

Cooking Time: 10 Minutes

Ingredients:

- 1 cup Drained and rinsed canned black beans
- ⅓ cup Pecan pieces
- ⅓ cup Rolled oats (not quick-cooking or steel-cut; gluten-free, if a concern)
- 2 tablespoons (or 1 small egg) Pasteurized egg substitute, such as Egg Beaters (gluten-free, if a concern)
- 2 teaspoons Red ketchup-like chili sauce, such as Heinz
- ¼ teaspoon Ground cumin
- ¼ teaspoon Dried oregano
- ¼ teaspoon Table salt
- ¼ teaspoon Ground black pepper
- Olive oil
- Olive oil spray

Directions:

1. Preheat the air fryer to 400°F.
2. Put the beans, pecans, oats, egg substitute or egg, chili sauce, cumin, oregano, salt, and pepper in a food processor. Cover and process to a coarse paste that will hold its shape like sugar-cookie dough, adding olive oil in 1-teaspoon increments to get the mixture to blend smoothly. The amount of olive oil is actually dependent on the internal moisture content of the beans and the oats. Figure on about 1 tablespoon (three 1-teaspoon additions) for the smaller batch, with proportional increases for the other batches. A little too much olive oil can't hurt, but a dry paste will fall apart as it cooks and a far-too-wet paste will stick to the basket.
3. Scrape down and remove the blade. Using clean, wet hands, form the paste into two 4-inch patties for the small batch, three 4-inch patties for the medium, or four 4-inch patties for the large batch, setting them one by one on a cutting board. Generously coat both sides of the patties with olive oil spray.
4. Set them in the basket in one layer. Air-fry undisturbed for 10 minutes, or until lightly browned and crisp at the edges.
5. Use a nonstick-safe spatula, and perhaps a flatware fork for balance, to transfer the burgers to a wire rack. Cool for 5 minutes before serving.

Salmon Burgers

Servings: 3

Cooking Time: 8 Minutes

Ingredients:

- 1 pound 2 ounces Skinless salmon fillet, preferably fattier Atlantic salmon
- 1½ tablespoons Minced chives or the green part of a scallion
- ½ cup Plain panko bread crumbs (gluten-free, if a concern)
- 1½ teaspoons Dijon mustard (gluten-free, if a concern)
- 1½ teaspoons Drained and rinsed capers, minced
- 1½ teaspoons Lemon juice
- ¼ teaspoon Table salt
- ¼ teaspoon Ground black pepper
- Vegetable oil spray

Directions:

1. Preheat the air fryer to 375°F .
2. Cut the salmon into pieces that will fit in a food processor. Cover and pulse until coarsely chopped. Add the chives and pulse to combine, until the fish is ground but not a paste. Scrape down and remove the blade. Scrape the salmon mixture into a bowl. Add the bread crumbs, mustard, capers, lemon juice, salt, and pepper. Stir gently until well combined.
3. Use clean and dry hands to form the mixture into two 5-inch patties for a small batch, three 5-inch patties for a medium batch, or four 5-inch patties for a large one.
4. Coat both sides of each patty with vegetable oil spray. Set them in the basket in one layer and air-fry undisturbed for 8 minutes, or until browned and an instant-read meat thermometer inserted into the center of a burger registers 145°F.
5. Use a nonstick-safe spatula, and perhaps a flatware fork for balance, to transfer the burgers to a wire rack. Cool for 2 or 3 minutes before serving.

Chicken Apple Brie Melt

Servings: 3

Cooking Time: 13 Minutes

Ingredients:

- 3 5- to 6-ounce boneless skinless chicken breasts
- Vegetable oil spray
- 1½ teaspoons Dried herbes de Provence
- 3 ounces Brie, rind removed, thinly sliced
- 6 Thin cored apple slices
- 3 French rolls (gluten-free, if a concern)
- 2 tablespoons Dijon mustard (gluten-free, if a concern)

Directions:

1. Preheat the air fryer to 375°F .
2. Lightly coat all sides of the chicken breasts with vegetable oil spray. Sprinkle the breasts evenly with the herbes de Provence.
3. When the machine is at temperature, set the breasts in the basket and air-fry undisturbed for 10 minutes.
4. Top the chicken breasts with the apple slices, then the cheese. Air-fry undisturbed for 2 minutes, or until the cheese is melty and bubbling.
5. Use a nonstick-safe spatula and kitchen tongs, for balance, to transfer the breasts to a cutting board. Set the rolls in the basket and air-fry for 1 minute to warm through. (Putting them in the machine without splitting them keeps the insides very soft while the outside gets a little crunchy.)
6. Transfer the rolls to the cutting board. Split them open lengthwise, then spread 1 teaspoon mustard on each cut side. Set a prepared chicken breast on the bottom of a roll and close with its top, repeating as necessary to make additional sandwiches. Serve warm.

Fish And Seafood Recipes

Lobster Tails With Lemon Garlic Butter

Servings: 2

Cooking Time: 5 Minutes

Ingredients:

- 4 ounces unsalted butter
- 1 tablespoon finely chopped lemon zest
- 1 clove garlic, thinly sliced
- 2 (6-ounce) lobster tails
- salt and freshly ground black pepper
- ½ cup white wine
- ½ lemon, sliced
- vegetable oil

Directions:

1. Start by making the lemon garlic butter. Combine the butter, lemon zest and garlic in a small saucepan. Melt and simmer the butter on the stovetop over the lowest possible heat while you prepare the lobster tails.
2. Prepare the lobster tails by cutting down the middle of the top of the shell. Crack the bottom shell by squeezing the sides of the lobster together so that you can access the lobster meat inside. Pull the lobster tail up out of the shell, but leave it attached at the base of the tail. Lay the lobster meat on top of the shell and season with salt and freshly ground black pepper. Pour a little of the lemon garlic butter on top of the lobster meat and transfer the lobster to the refrigerator so that the butter solidifies a little.
3. Pour the white wine into the air fryer drawer and add the lemon slices. Preheat the air fryer to 400°F for 5 minutes.
4. Transfer the lobster tails to the air fryer basket. Air-fry at 370° for 5 minutes, brushing more butter on halfway through cooking. (Add a minute or two if your lobster tail is more than 6-ounces.) Remove and serve with more butter for dipping or drizzling.

Easy Scallops With Lemon Butter

Servings:3

Cooking Time: 4 Minutes

Ingredients:

- 1 tablespoon Olive oil
- 2 teaspoons Minced garlic
- 1 teaspoon Finely grated lemon zest
- ½ teaspoon Red pepper flakes
- ¼ teaspoon Table salt
- 1 pound Sea scallops
- 3 tablespoons Butter, melted
- 1½ tablespoons Lemon juice

Directions:

1. Preheat the air fryer to 400°F.
2. Gently stir the olive oil, garlic, lemon zest, red pepper flakes, and salt in a bowl. Add the scallops and stir very gently until they are evenly and well coated.
3. When the machine is at temperature, arrange the scallops in a single layer in the basket. Some may touch. Air-fry undisturbed for 4 minutes, or until the scallops are opaque and firm.
4. While the scallops cook, stir the melted butter and lemon juice in a serving bowl. When the scallops are ready, pour them from the basket into this bowl. Toss well before serving.

Black Cod With Grapes, Fennel, Pecans And Kale

Servings: 2

Cooking Time: 15 Minutes

Ingredients:

- 2 (6- to 8-ounce) fillets of black cod (or sablefish)
- salt and freshly ground black pepper
- olive oil
- 1 cup grapes, halved
- 1 small bulb fennel, sliced ¼-inch thick
- ½ cup pecans
- 3 cups shredded kale
- 2 teaspoons white balsamic vinegar or white wine vinegar
- 2 tablespoons extra virgin olive oil

Directions:

1. Preheat the air fryer to 400°F.
2. Season the cod fillets with salt and pepper and drizzle, brush or spray a little olive oil on top. Place the fish, presentation side up (skin side down), into the air fryer basket. Air-fry for 10 minutes.
3. When the fish has finished cooking, remove the fillets to a side plate and loosely tent with foil to rest.
4. Toss the grapes, fennel and pecans in a bowl with a drizzle of olive oil and season with salt and pepper. Add the grapes, fennel and pecans to the air fryer basket and air-fry for 5 minutes at 400°F, shaking the basket once during the cooking time.
5. Transfer the grapes, fennel and pecans to a bowl with the kale. Dress the kale with the balsamic vinegar and olive oil, season to taste with salt and pepper and serve along side the cooked fish.

Coconut Shrimp

Servings: 4

Cooking Time: 12 Minutes

Ingredients:

- 1 pound large shrimp (about 16 to 20), peeled and de-veined
- ½ cup flour
- salt and freshly ground black pepper
- 2 egg whites
- ½ cup fine breadcrumbs
- ½ cup shredded unsweetened coconut
- zest of one lime
- ½ teaspoon salt
- ⅛ to ¼ teaspoon ground cayenne pepper
- vegetable or canola oil
- sweet chili sauce or duck sauce (for serving)

Directions:

1. Set up a dredging station. Place the flour in a shallow dish and season well with salt and freshly ground black pepper. Whisk the egg whites in a second shallow dish. In a third shallow dish, combine the breadcrumbs, coconut, lime zest, salt and cayenne pepper.
2. Preheat the air fryer to 400°F.
3. Dredge each shrimp first in the flour, then dip it in the egg mixture, and finally press it into the breadcrumb-coconut mixture to coat all sides. Place the breaded shrimp on a plate or baking sheet and spray both sides with vegetable oil.
4. Air-fry the shrimp in two batches, being sure not to over-crowd the basket. Air-fry for 5 minutes, turning the shrimp over for the last minute or two. Repeat with the second batch of shrimp.
5. Lower the temperature of the air fryer to 340°F. Return the first batch of shrimp to the air fryer basket with the second batch and air-fry for an additional 2 minutes, just to re-heat everything.
6. Serve with sweet chili sauce, duck sauce or just eat them plain!

Shrimp & Grits

Servings: 4

Cooking Time: 5 Minutes

Ingredients:

- 1 pound raw shelled shrimp, deveined (26–30 count or smaller)
- Marinade
- 2 tablespoons lemon juice
- 2 tablespoons Worcestershire sauce
- 1 tablespoon olive oil
- 1 teaspoon Old Bay Seasoning
- ½ teaspoon hot sauce
- Grits
- ¾ cup quick cooking grits (not instant)
- 3 cups water
- ½ teaspoon salt
- 1 tablespoon butter
- ½ cup chopped green bell pepper
- ½ cup chopped celery
- ½ cup chopped onion
- ½ teaspoon oregano
- ¼ teaspoon Old Bay Seasoning
- 2 ounces sharp Cheddar cheese, grated

Directions:

1. Stir together all marinade ingredients. Pour marinade over shrimp and set aside.
2. For grits, heat water and salt to boil in saucepan on stovetop. Stir in grits, lower heat to medium-low, and cook about 5minutes or until thick and done.
3. Place butter, bell pepper, celery, and onion in air fryer baking pan. Cook at 390°F for 2minutes and stir. Cook 6 or 7minutes longer, until crisp tender.
4. Add oregano and 1 teaspoon Old Bay to cooked vegetables. Stir in grits and cheese and cook at 390°F for 1 minute. Stir and cook 1 to 2minutes longer to melt cheese.
5. Remove baking pan from air fryer. Cover with plate to keep warm while shrimp cooks.
6. Drain marinade from shrimp. Place shrimp in air fryer basket and cook at 360°F for 3minutes. Stir or shake basket. Cook 2 more minutes, until done.
7. To serve, spoon grits onto plates and top with shrimp.

Tuna Nuggets In Hoisin Sauce

Servings: 4

Cooking Time: 7 Minutes

Ingredients:

- ½ cup hoisin sauce
- 2 tablespoons rice wine vinegar
- 2 teaspoons sesame oil
- 1 teaspoon garlic powder
- 2 teaspoons dried lemongrass
- ¼ teaspoon red pepper flakes
- ½ small onion, quartered and thinly sliced
- 8 ounces fresh tuna, cut into 1-inch cubes
- cooking spray
- 3 cups cooked jasmine rice

Directions:

1. Mix the hoisin sauce, vinegar, sesame oil, and seasonings together.
2. Stir in the onions and tuna nuggets.
3. Spray air fryer baking pan with nonstick spray and pour in tuna mixture.
4. Cook at 390°F for 3minutes. Stir gently.
5. Cook 2minutes and stir again, checking for doneness. Tuna should be barely cooked through, just beginning to flake and still very moist. If necessary, continue cooking and stirring in 1-minute intervals until done.
6. Serve warm over hot jasmine rice.

Coconut Jerk Shrimp

Servings:3

Cooking Time: 8 Minutes

Ingredients:

- 1 Large egg white(s)
- 1 teaspoon Purchased or homemade jerk dried seasoning blend (see the headnote)
- ¾ cup Plain panko bread crumbs (gluten-free, if a concern)
- ¾ cup Unsweetened shredded coconut
- 12 Large shrimp (20–25 per pound), peeled and deveined
- Coconut oil spray

Directions:

1. Preheat the air fryer to 375°F .
2. Whisk the egg white(s) and seasoning blend in a bowl until foamy. Add the shrimp and toss well to coat evenly.
3. Mix the bread crumbs and coconut on a dinner plate until well combined. Use kitchen tongs to pick up a shrimp, letting the excess egg white mixture slip back into the rest. Set the shrimp in the bread-crumb mixture. Turn several times to coat evenly and thoroughly. Set on a cutting board and continue coating the remainder of the shrimp.
4. Lightly coat all the shrimp on both sides with the coconut oil spray. Set them in the basket in one layer with as much space between them as possible. (You can even stand some up along the basket's wall in some models.) Air-fry undisturbed for 6 minutes, or until the coating is lightly browned. If the air fryer is at 360°F, you may need to add 2 minutes to the cooking time.
5. Use clean kitchen tongs to transfer the shrimp to a wire rack. Cool for only a minute or two before serving.

Shrimp "scampi"

Servings:4

Cooking Time: 5 Minutes

Ingredients:

- 1½ pounds Large shrimp (20–25 per pound), peeled and deveined
- ¼ cup Olive oil
- 2 tablespoons Minced garlic
- 1 teaspoon Dried oregano
- Up to 1 teaspoon Red pepper flakes
- ½ teaspoon Table salt
- 2 tablespoons White balsamic vinegar (see here)

Directions:

1. Preheat the air fryer to 400°F.
2. Stir the shrimp, olive oil, garlic, oregano, red pepper flakes, and salt in a large bowl until the shrimp are well coated.
3. When the machine is at temperature, transfer the shrimp to the basket. They will overlap and even sit on top of each other. Air-fry for 5 minutes, tossing and rearranging the shrimp twice to make sure the covered surfaces are exposed, until pink and firm.
4. Pour the contents of the basket into a serving bowl. Pour the vinegar over the shrimp while hot and toss to coat.

Almond-crusted Fish

Servings: 4

Cooking Time: 10 Minutes

Ingredients:

- 4 4-ounce fish fillets
- ¾ cup breadcrumbs
- ¼ cup sliced almonds, crushed
- 2 tablespoons lemon juice
- ⅛ teaspoon cayenne
- salt and pepper
- ¾ cup flour
- 1 egg, beaten with 1 tablespoon water
- oil for misting or cooking spray

Directions:

1. Split fish fillets lengthwise down the center to create 8 pieces.
2. Mix breadcrumbs and almonds together and set aside.
3. Mix the lemon juice and cayenne together. Brush on all sides of fish.
4. Season fish to taste with salt and pepper.
5. Place the flour on a sheet of wax paper.
6. Roll fillets in flour, dip in egg wash, and roll in the crumb mixture.
7. Mist both sides of fish with oil or cooking spray.
8. Spray air fryer basket and lay fillets inside.
9. Cook at 390°F for 5minutes, turn fish over, and cook for an additional 5minutes or until fish is done and flakes easily.

Fried Scallops

Servings:3

Cooking Time: 6 Minutes

Ingredients:

- ½ cup All-purpose flour or tapioca flour
- 1 Large egg(s), well beaten
- 2 cups Corn flake crumbs (gluten-free, if a concern)
- Up to 2 teaspoons Cayenne
- 1 teaspoon Celery seeds
- 1 teaspoon Table salt
- 1 pound Sea scallops
- Vegetable oil spray

Directions:

1. Preheat the air fryer to 400°F.
2. Set up and fill three shallow soup plates or small pie plates on your counter: one for the flour; one for the beaten egg(s); and one for the corn flake crumbs, stirred with the cayenne, celery seeds, and salt until well combined.
3. One by one, dip a scallop in the flour, turning it every way to coat it thoroughly. Gently shake off any excess flour, then dip the scallop in the egg(s), turning it again to coat all sides. Let any excess egg slip back into the rest, then set the scallop in the corn flake mixture. Turn it several times, pressing gently to get an even coating on the scallop all around. Generously coat the scallop with vegetable oil spray, then set it aside on a cutting board. Coat the remaining scallops in the same way.
4. Set the scallops in the basket with as much air space between them as possible. They should not touch. Air-fry undisturbed for 6 minutes, or until lightly browned and firm.
5. Use kitchen tongs to gently transfer the scallops to a wire rack. Cool for only a minute or two before serving.

Lightning Source UK Ltd.
Milton Keynes UK
UKHW051626230123
415821UK00015B/574

9 781802 448306